The Longest Journey To Goodbye

A Caregiver's Story of the Ravages of Young Onset Alzheimer's Disease and Related Dementias

By
Frederick Russo

Dedication

This book is dedicated to my wife, Elizabeth, my sons, Fred and David, and their families, Theresa Franklin and Carol Russo.

Also, Connie Wasserman and the Sid Jacobson Center, the staff of the dementia wing of Bristal Assisted Living, East Meadow, and my support group.

Quotation

"All right," said the cat; and at this time it vanished quite slowly, beginning with the end of the tail, and ending with the grin, which remained some time after the rest of it had gone. "Well I've often seen a cat without a grin," thought Alice; " but a grin without a cat! It's the most curious thing I ever saw in all my life!"

Alice and the Cheshire Cat, from Alice's Adventures in Wonderland, by Lewis Carroll.

Table of Contents

Prologue

Alzheimer's disease affects over six million Americans today. Young Onset Alzheimer's affects 10% of all Alzheimer's victims. People with Young Onset Alzheimer's are between the ages of 35 to 60 years of age. Previously, it was thought that Alzheimer's and related dementias attacked people in their 70s and 80s. It was so common that we used to just call all these related dementias "senility."

This is the story of a caregiver learning to struggle with the ravages of dementia as related to his wife. The reader will immediately see the total ineptitude and lack of knowledge that I, as a caregiver, had at the beginning to middle of this journey. Everything I learned was hard won and always as a result of, or in response to situations as they developed.

In the beginning, I was basically clueless about how to deal with this and completely overwhelmed by the magnitude of the undertaking. Denial and anger were my two most common emotional states. Hopefully, you will see the evolution of a caregiver (in dealing with this disease) to a point where he has finally accepted his role and has become quite good at it.

It is in the hope that future readers may benefit from my story, the knowledge I gained along the way, and as a tribute to my wife, that this story is written.

Chapter One:
The Early Years

I have been a caregiver for my wife, Elizabeth, who probably contracted the disease in her early forties but was undiagnosed for more than 15 years. It was undiagnosed because of the way the disease manifested itself.

Elizabeth and I met at college. She was majoring in English and was determined to be a writer and a poet. I was majoring in history and economics and was thinking of either going into the Peace Corps or law school. We met at a school dance, which neither of us wanted to go to. Her parents forced her to go, and my fraternity brothers persuaded me to be at the dance because it was the first week of the school term, and it was an opportunity to talk to freshmen and invite them to rush to your fraternity. I looked across the dance floor and noticed a beautiful girl looking as forlorn as me. I could tell she didn't want to be there any more than I did.

So, I went up to her and introduced myself by asking a really dumb opening question, but when you're young and awkward, it's hard not to be nervous. I asked if she was going to be a teacher, get married, and quit teaching after the guy started making big bucks. I stupidly thought that it sounded impressive and funny. She got mad and said in an angry voice that she had no interest in marriage and just wanted to be a writer. I apologized, and we talked about her favorite authors, James Joyce, T.S. Elliot, Dylan Thomas, and Emily Dickinson. We spent hours on the phone talking about everything.

Our mothers would threaten us by saying that we were going to have to pay the phone bills since we were dominating the phone line. She was my best friend, and there was nothing that we couldn't talk about. We kept nothing from each other, including times with other dates. We had decided that since neither of us had much dating experience, it wasn't fair to either of us not to explore and see if we were missing out. Maybe we would find someone we like better. We were willing to take that chance.

After about a year of exploration, we admitted to ourselves that it was a waste of time; we found ourselves talking about the horrible other dates and laughing at their foolishness. We decided to give up that venture. We were *"soulmates,"* and searching further was useless. We dated through all of college and through two and a half years of my Law School.

The Vietnam War was on, and we wanted to marry before I could be drafted.

After graduation, I got a job as an attorney with the federal government, giving up my idea of going into the Peace Corps while she was working as a buyer in a big New York City department store while still pursuing a writing career. We had a good married life with two children, great friends, and a house in the suburbs. We were living the American dream.

We were very artsy and had artsy friends. We were very educated liberals and scholastics living the good life with friends who were professors, teachers, scientists, mathematicians, etc., a very cultured group of young professionals. We thought our lives were as good as it gets. We worked hard and partied hard. We lived in this idyll into our early forties when things changed abruptly. That is when the disease began, though no one would know it for many years.

At first, the disease manifested as a personality change. At age forty-five, she was becoming more reclusive, not enjoying the life we had built, and much more emotionally detached. I thought it could be a change of life or clinical depression. I tried to get her to see a doctor. By that time, she was a "born-again Christian" and had a pat answer for a doctor's visit.

She was proud of saying, "Doctor Jesus would heal her." She didn't need any doctors.

When pressed, she would strike back, "Why are you all picking on me? There's nothing wrong with me; there's something wrong with you."

She also stopped cooking by that time. When questioned, she had a very clever answer, one that would deflect your thinking away from what I, many years later, learned was the real problem (that she was afraid she forgot how to cook and if she tried and failed, her secret would be out in the open and action would have been taken—her pride and vanity would not permit this to happen).

So, she cleverly said, "I don't cook anymore, but I've been there and done that. Why don't you cook? We both work. Why should I be the only one that cooks?"

I had to admit she had a strong point, one hard to argue with. So I suggested that we eat out after work. We did this routine of picking up our sons after work and going to a local diner or restaurant.

This worked for about one year. Then, the boys rebelled. They said they were tired of eating out; they would rather stay home and have "mac and cheese" than join us for dinner every night.

By that time, I had had it, too. I didn't want to eat out every night, either. So, I told the boys I would make us dinner on weeknights if they would join us for a family meal on Sundays. I told them I would take their mother out to dinner on Fridays and Saturdays, and the rest of the nights, we would "eat in." This seemed to be an acceptable compromise, and it lasted for a very long time.

Meanwhile, she was developing strange behavior patterns. On weeknights, when I cooked dinner, my wife would not eat with us. She would carefully portion out the leftovers from our eating out nights (Fri, Sat, and Sunday) and microwave a portion. She would go into another room, watch TV, and eat her dinner alone. She would always ask for a take-home bag for her food, and she would eat only about a third of her meal so that she would have 2/3rds left for the rest of the following week. This way, she would never run out of food and would never be challenged to cook anything. Of course, it took me a very long time to figure out what she was doing and why.

At first, I thought she was being unbelievably heartless and cruel—how could a mother suddenly not want to be with her own children? I had a lot of resentment and not a clue that she was getting sick with a deadly disease. I comforted my resentment by telling myself that this was probably a "change of life" and would disappear in a few years.

My youngest son said, "Dad, Mom doesn't go out with you to eat; she goes out to shop for food."

Of course, why hadn't I seen this? She was hiding the fact that she couldn't cook any longer. By taking home her food from the restaurants we frequented on weekends, she had enough food to feed herself for the week by simply microwaving the leftovers.

In the meantime, there were other strange behavior patterns developing in the form of inappropriate laughter and a complete lack of social discretion. Having no training in medicine or psychology, I was ill-equipped to diagnose my wife's new strange behavior. I was also so in denial, and I found myself always making excuses for her new bizarre behavior.

She would laugh at anything and everything and say anything without a thought as to whether it might hurt another or how it might be received. In a restaurant, she would announce that she needed to go to the bathroom and tell us about the bodily function involved. I would constantly be telling her that no one wanted to hear what she was doing in the bathroom, and it was sufficient to just leave it at just the "I am going to the bathroom" statement. Another time we went to the wedding of our very good friend's son. It wasn't long before my wife cornered the bride and, in casual conversation, asked her if she was *pregnant or just fat*. The bride was so mortified that she hid in the bathroom and cried.

At work, in a family business, and with a company that had a large repair and service component, she angered our customers with statements like, "God broke the equipment because you haven't paid the balance of your bill."

After a while and with mounting customer complaints about her strange, rude, and confrontational behavior, we decided to retire her from the family business, giving her bookkeeping work to do at home while keeping duplicate financial files on the computer at the office (her bookkeeping being just a way to keep her busy and feeling useful). But this didn't occur till much later.

She was also having problems with language. My wife had been a published poet and had the command of a huge vocabulary. When she started to show changes, she stopped initiating any conversation and would answer only specific questions put to her with very terse replies. Her vocabulary would slip from two hundred thousand plus words to about twenty-five words and, toward the end, from twenty-five words down to nothing.

Chapter Two:
Starting to Forget

With our friends and in social situations, I did the cooking and the entertaining.

There came a time when I invited our very good friends whom we had known from college days over for dinner. I, of course, did the cooking but asked my wife to mix the salad, which she agreed to do. While I was preparing the lobster, I asked if anyone would like some wine before dinner. They said yes, and I asked my wife, who was mixing the salad at that moment, to bring me a corkscrew. She blithely replied, ***"What's a corkscrew?"***

What followed was a deafening silence. She went to the bathroom, and both our friends approached me and insisted that I take my wife to a doctor. They said I had been excusing her behavior too long and that I must see that her strange behavior had become so obvious to them that they couldn't understand how I didn't see it. They had known both of us since we were college kids in our twenties and had painfully watched one of us deteriorate to this point. They reminded me that my wife had been a gourmet chef and could never have forgotten the name of such a simple kitchen utensil (as a corkscrew). They told me they could no longer sit silently and watch any longer and insisted that I take action. I promised that I would, and thus began the middle stage of the saga of this illness.

I approached the Alzheimer's Association and Long Island Alzheimer's Foundation for advice and resources. I didn't know where to begin looking for help and felt positively overwhelmed by the enormity of the problem. I learned that there was a weekly support group meeting in Mineola, and I started going there for counsel.

In those days, most of the participants in the group were children of parents with dementia. I felt no bond with this group as I was dealing with the loss of a wife, not a parent. My problems were so vastly different from dealing with a parent (except for the basics of caregiving). In my case, it was the loss of a best friend, a lover, creating a huge hole in one's life that could not be easily filled or fixed.

Eventually, I found a group called **"Well Spouse,"** which dealt with spouses of persons with terminal illnesses such as cancer, MS, etc. I was the lone group member whose spouse had a terminal dementia disease, but at least the group's focus was dealing with the loss of a spouse and not parents (with an illness).

During that time, I heard an ad on the radio for Mt. Sinai Hospital in Manhattan. They were starting a clinical trial of new drugs that might prolong the progress of the disease and allow the lucid periods to last longer. We visited Mt Sinai once a week, and all observatory reports were coming up normal.

The doctors told me that Elizabeth had great concentration powers and that the written tests for cognitive ability were well within the normal range. They had no explanation for her strange behavior patterns (which were becoming worse and more frequent), nor did they observe them because she was careful to hide them from the doctors in her weekly meetings. I was referred to immunologists, cardiovascular specialists, and numerous others where, after extensive testing, she was still found to be in the range of normal.

Chapter Three:
The Middle Years

At that time, my youngest son, David, was going to college in Philadelphia and would occasionally come home on weekends. I was always thrilled and honored to know he loved us and felt comfortable spending a few weekends at home rather than with his college chums in some "Philly hotspot."

One weekend, when he came home, he and I were sitting in the kitchen talking when my wife came in. When she saw her son, she didn't say hello. She just asked why he was home and why did he move the salt shaker from its usual spot (and put it back). I couldn't believe that, as a mother, she wasn't overjoyed at the surprise visit. She wasn't! Instead, she was annoyed that he was altering the routine. I was devastated.

I had read about the Alzheimer's research being conducted at the University at Pittsburg, PA, where, with a special dye injected into the patient and with a PET scan, they were able to see amyloid plaque building up in areas of the brain associated with behavior and memory. The researchers thought that the plaque might be a cause of Alzheimer's and related dementias. When I mentioned this to her doctors, they indicated that they had heard of the study but did not show a willingness to submit my wife to this kind of testing. When I pushed to have her tested, I was told that no insurance company plan covered the cost and that if I insisted, they would do it for me on a private pay basis.

I fortunately decided that the test must be done, and I told her doctor that I would pay for the test "out of pocket," but I insisted that the test be performed. Several days later, when the results of the test came in, the PET scan clearly showed that the frontal lobes of the brain were significantly atrophied.

Suddenly, things started to make sense. The frontal lobes were the seat of linguistic cognition, and she had lost a tremendous amount of her prodigious vocabulary by then. Now I understood why she was mostly silent, only speaking to answer direct, clear questions and never initiating any conversation.

The frontal lobes also control the brain's filters for appropriate behavior and inappropriate laughter. She managed to fit all these symptoms. Now, I understood where the strange behavior was coming from. Now, I saw that her annoyance with her son for moving a kitchen item was caused by the rupture of routine, which took the place of having to remember something.

Chapter Four:
Driving the Car

In early 2004, I became increasingly anxious about my wife's ability to drive her car. I wasn't confident that she had sufficient judgment or requisite motor skills to continue to drive her car safely. She was so strong in her confidence that there was nothing wrong with her. She was defensive and combative. She said that she was being picked on by everybody, that she was a great driver, and that she would never consider giving up her driver's license. It was almost as if the license had become the last vestige of her pride, the last area of her life that she felt she could control. Everything else was slipping away from her, but she was still good at driving. Taking her car away from her was like cutting off her legs. She wouldn't give up her license without a war.

During this time, she was having episodes with the police, which, like a little girl, she thought was hilarious. I got a call one day from Winthrop Hospital, saying that they had my wife in the emergency room. My heart jumped when I heard those words. I caught my breath and managed to ask if she was okay.

The nurse told me, "Yes, we are just holding her for observation. The police brought her here because when they pulled her over for an illegal turn, she seemed to be acting irrationally, and they thought she might be on drugs. She was laughing at all the police's questions while they tried to interrogate her. They decided to impound her car and drive her to the hospital, where she is now and where she will stay until you come to discharge her."

I was flabbergasted! I should have seen this coming, but I was still in denial (the problem wasn't as bad as it seemed to others), and I wasn't making the best decisions. When I picked her up, she was laughing and in great spirits, as if the whole thing was a big joke and great fun. We argued that night about her giving up the car to no avail.

Every day, she would get in her car and drive somewhere. Usually, it was to the office, to church, to the stationers where she would buy her cigarettes, or to one of her friend's homes. All of these trips were routine and frequently taken. She always drove to each of her routine visits on the same exact roads, highways, and streets. She never varied. I knew this because when she was driving with me, she would always question me as to why I took this route and not another (meaning the one she always took). She seemed to get very uncomfortable when I deviated from her accustomed routes. This point was to be driven home to me in the very near future. It was late summer when I came home to an empty house. My sons had moved out and married, and the family sheepdog (my constant companion) had died a year earlier.

At first, I didn't think much of it; I just figured she was out at one of her usual places and would be home shortly. I was going to have a quick dinner and then go out to play chess at the chess club. I started to worry after I had finished my dinner. She still wasn't home because, as a creature of habit, she was always home by nightfall. I made some calls; nobody had seen her or knew her whereabouts. After another hour had passed, I decided to call the police and report her as missing.

Within a half hour, a patrolman and a detective showed up at my door, asked questions, and filled out paperwork. I also called my sons, and they came over to help me. I was frantic. The detective explained to me that when dealing with people with dementia if they are walkers, they will walk till they drop or find their way back home again. He said he knew a case where a person from Nassau County had been found the next morning on a street corner in Queens (another county). He said when they are in a car, they drive it until they run out of gas or find their way home. When I told him that she would never run out of gas because she had a gas card, he told me that he was going to expand the search. He said she could be on I-95 driving anywhere from Maine to Florida!

Now, I was stunned again. I finally realized how serious her driving problem was. I vowed that if we found her alive, I would do all in my power to wrest the car from her and then figure out how to deal with her driver's license. I remember the winter before when I came home and was met by my neighbor who told me my wife was in the hospital because she was trying to get into the car when she fell on the ice. Instead of trying to get up or crawling back to the house or even the grass where she might have better footing, she just sat there until the neighbor called the ambulance. When I got to the hospital, they told me they were treating her for hypothermia. I was asking myself, *How did I let things get so out of hand? Why didn't I act sooner?*

At about 9 pm, as we contemplated her possible whereabouts and filled out all the paperwork, my wife came waltzing in, happy and laughing. When we questioned her, she said she had gone to church, but when she tried to come home by her usual route, there was a construction crew who had closed Post Ave (a street not more than a half mile from our home), and she didn't know how to get home.

We had lived in Westbury for 30+ years, and she had known all the side streets, but now, with her routine being interrupted just slightly, just infinitesimally, she would become inexorably lost. It was shocking to see how far she had regressed and also what an apologist for her I had become; that I had permitted myself to be unaware of how grave a danger she was becoming. I went to bed that night exhausted and shaken.

Tomorrow morning, I will figure out how to get the car from her, I thought.

I tried several times to talk to my wife, Elizabeth, about giving up her license, but again, to no avail, so I took a different course of action. I read some articles on dementia where it was suggested that you could never win by arguing with the Alzheimer's patient.

Logic will not work, and even if you convince them you are right, five minutes later, you have to revisit it all over again as if the first conversation never happened because, in their minds, it never did. Until you understand this basic fact, you cannot deal with caring for a person with Alzheimer's at all. So, when an argument starts, we learn to try distraction, deflection, and, yes, deception.

This time, instead of arguing with Elizabeth about giving up her license, I did two things: I asked a neighbor to report her erratic driving behavior to the motor vehicle department, and I disconnected the battery in her car. The first is important because nobody in the family needs to be the "bad guy" (it's the Motor Vehicle Bureau), and secondly, the car doesn't work anymore, so it needs to go in for repair. The tactic worked to perfection.

Two weeks after she was reported, she received a certified letter requesting her presence at a hearing to determine her continuing ability to drive a car. She ignored the notice and refused to go to the hearing. I believe that in her heart, she knew she would never pass the test. Also, I called the Audi dealership and asked them to tow the car away. I told my wife that the car was to be fixed and returned, but I told the dealer to sell the car. She asked a couple of times about the status of the repairs, and I told her the parts were on order from Germany.

After a couple of weeks, she never asked again, and the problem of her driving went away without so much as an argument. It was over, and it was that easy! Then, the next coup was to wrest the driver's license from her. That was just as easily accomplished. I took her to the Motor Vehicle Department and told her we were going to get a new, updated license. We, in fact, got a new New York State driver's identification certificate (a picture ID) that looks exactly like a NY driver's license. She was content, and that ended the driving saga completely.

Chapter Five: Dangerous Behavior

From about early 2001, she started exhibiting dangerous behavior patterns. She would treat the home heating system as if it were a toy contraption to play with and abuse. When she felt cold, she would turn the thermostat to 90 degrees, wait till it got warm enough, and then turn it way down to 70 degrees after she felt comfortable. I told her repeatedly that this could put a terrible strain on an old system and possibly cause the furnace to explode.

She refused to believe it because this was exactly the way she handled her car heater. When she started the car in cold weather, she would put the heat up to "max" and lower it when she felt warm. She was sure that by turning the thermostat to "max," the car (and, therefore, the home) would heat faster.

As many times as I told my wife, Elizabeth, that the car would not begin to heat until the motor was hot and that no amount of playing with the thermostat would make any difference, she was convinced that her method would defy the principles of physics and make the car (and therefore the home) warm up faster. After innumerable arguments that drove me crazy, I finally had to resort to placing locked plastic covers over all the thermostats in our home. After that, she looked at the covers and laughed; she didn't argue, and the whole thing was forgotten.

Another dangerous habit of Elizabeth's was that she preferred to throw things down a flight of stairs rather than carry them down the stairs. In the late 1990s, Elizabeth started to exhibit a childish behavior pattern that is usually trained out before adulthood through parenting.

Elizabeth started to enjoy throwing things down the staircase. She would seem to take great pleasure in her accomplishment. She would stand at the top of the stairwell and laugh at the suitcase plummeting down the stairs, knocking pictures off walls, and bouncing off the door at the bottom. It didn't seem to bother her that she was destroying property as well as her suitcase. No matter how many times we have discussed this behavior as unacceptable, it will be repeated with no memory of any prior discussions.

By this time, I was beginning to realize that her retention span for instruction or conversation was about five minutes and that every five minutes, it was a new conversation.

One time in 2004, we went food shopping at the supermarket. We bought all the usual weekly food supplies, and she said she needed washing detergent for the clothes washer, so we bought some. When we arrived home, we started to put things away, and suddenly, I heard this tremendous crash. Elizabeth was standing at the top of the stairs, looking satisfied and satisfied at what she had done.

I went over to look, and to my horror, she had just thrown a bottle of liquid laundry detergent down the stairs. Thank God it hadn't broken, but what if it had? My mind raced as I clearly saw all the suds on the basement floor as I tried to clean it up, and the more water I used, the more suds would be produced. Even though it didn't happen, the thought that, but for dumb luck, it should have happened shook me to the core.

I became suddenly furious, and I grabbed my wife, pinned her up against a wall, and shook her violently, screaming, "Why did you do this?"

Her only reply was, "Why are you screaming at me? Why aren't you nice anymore, and why are you so mean?"

I started to tremble! I realized that I was now out of control. Part of me wanted to kill her; I was so furious, and part of me was feeling guilty for the anger, realizing that she was sick and could not help herself. Thus started a period where I would feel only two emotions: **"Anger and Guilt."** They would prove to be a toxic cocktail that would eventually bring me, the devoted caregiver, into crisis.

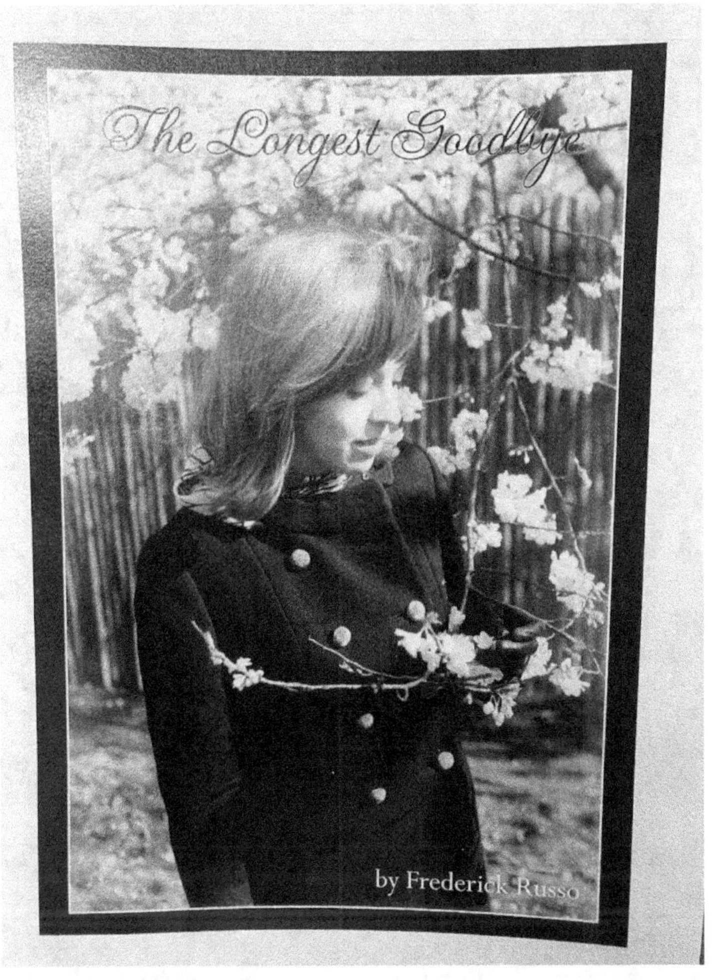

Cherry blossom time at botanic gardens 1967.

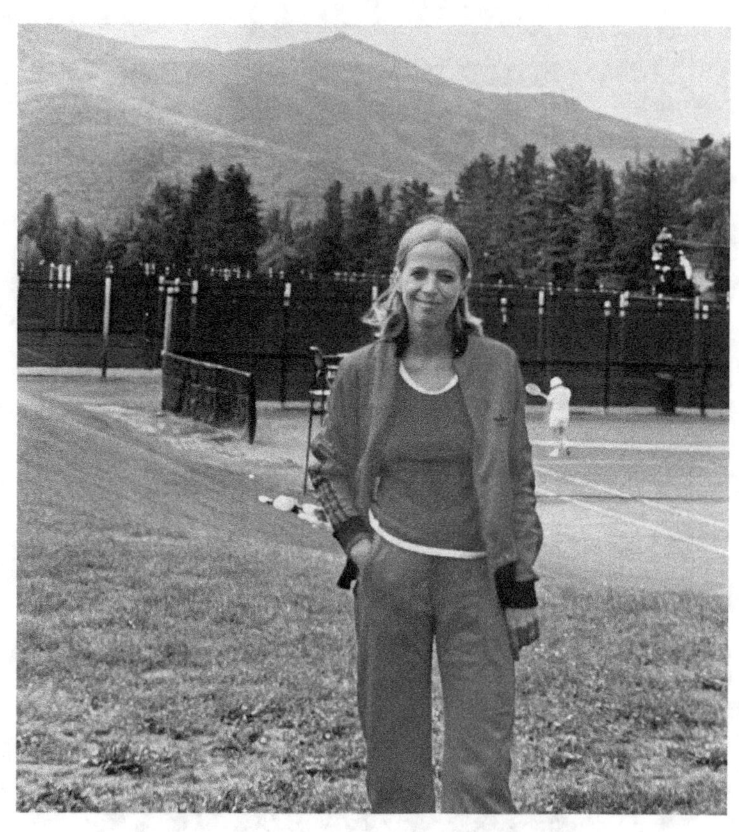

Elizabeth at tennis camp in New Hampshire 1977.

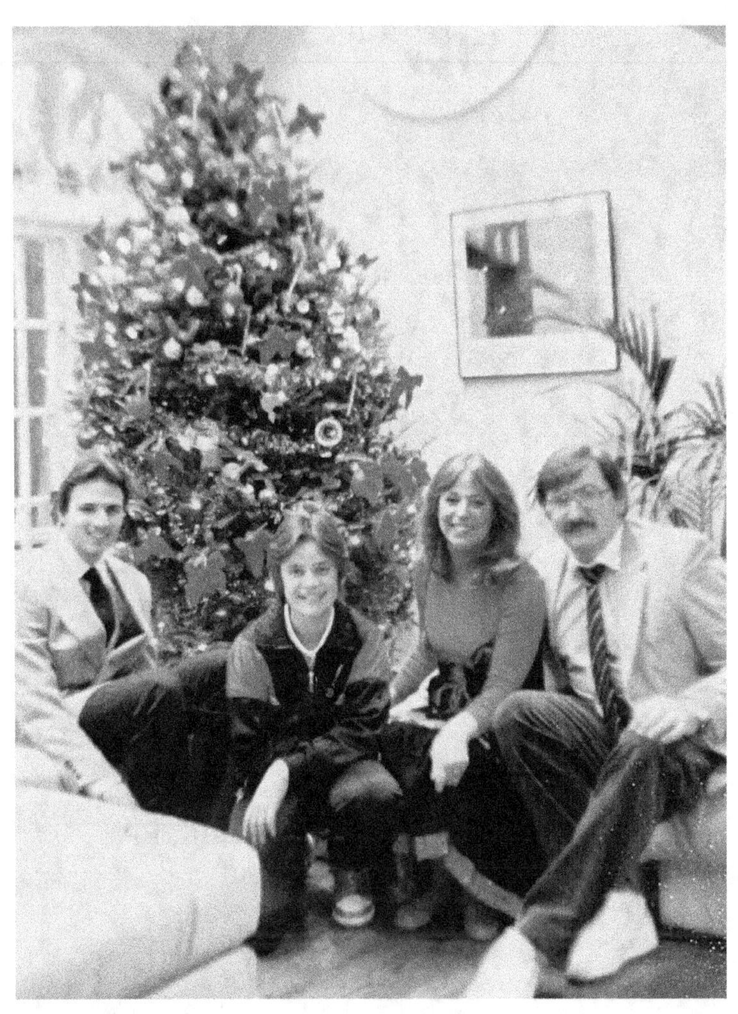

Christmas at home 1985.

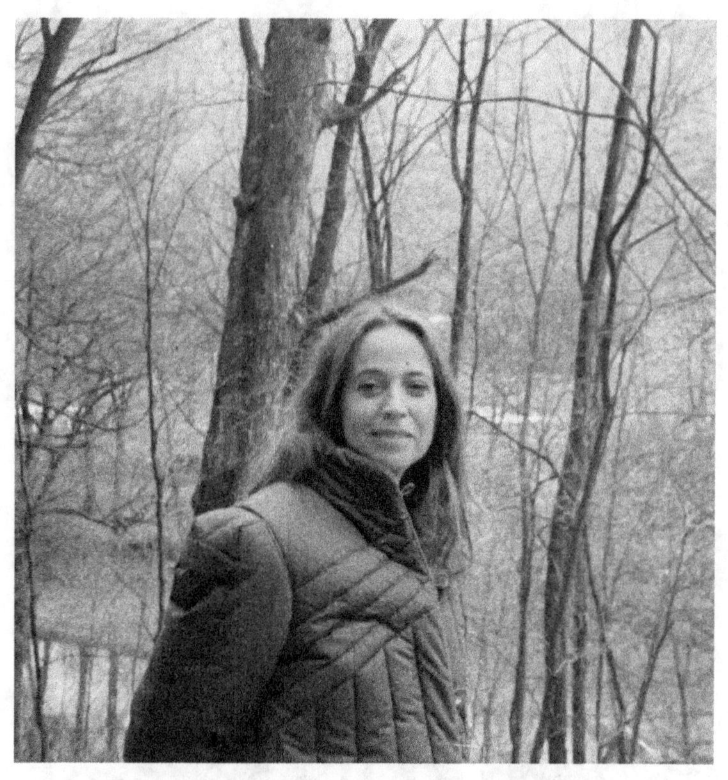

Hiking on the Appalachian trail, PA.

1985.

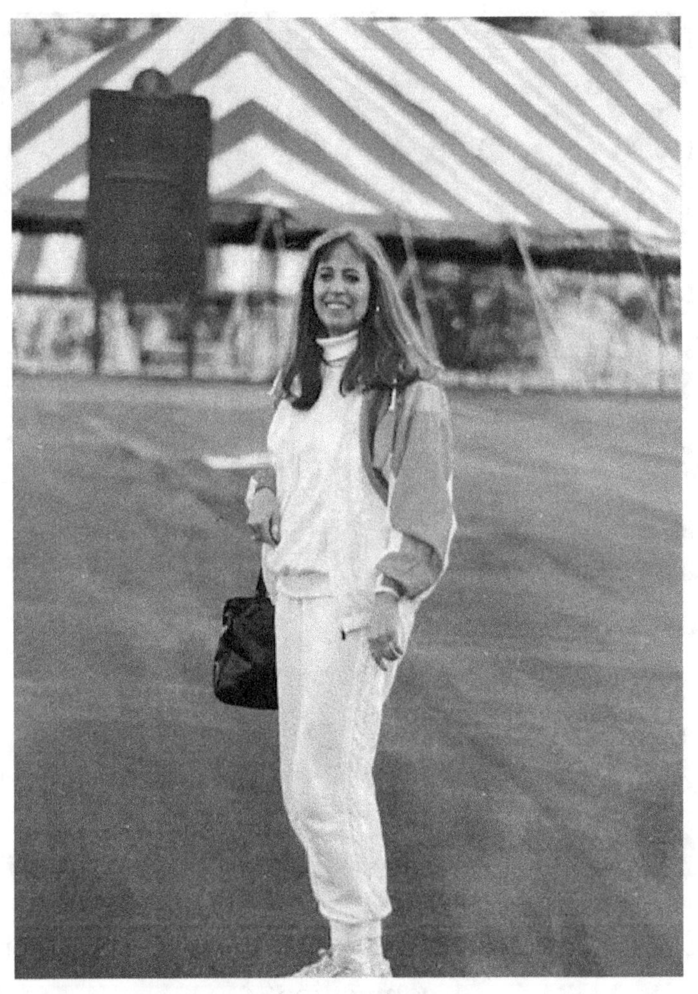

Fall balloon festival 1988.

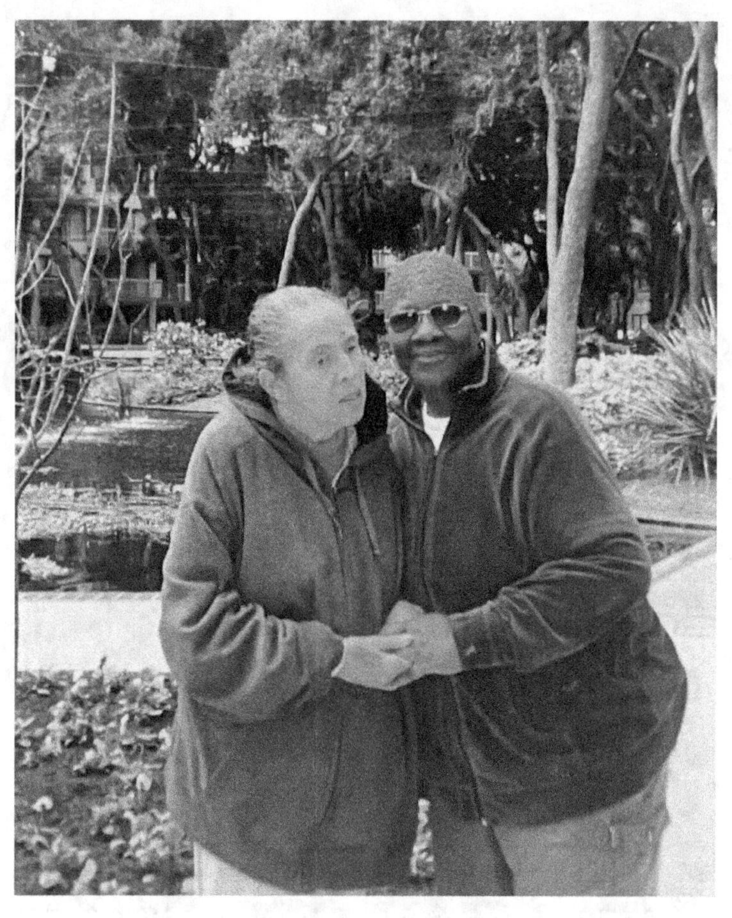

Elizabeth at Hilton Head 2007 with Theresa, her
companion.

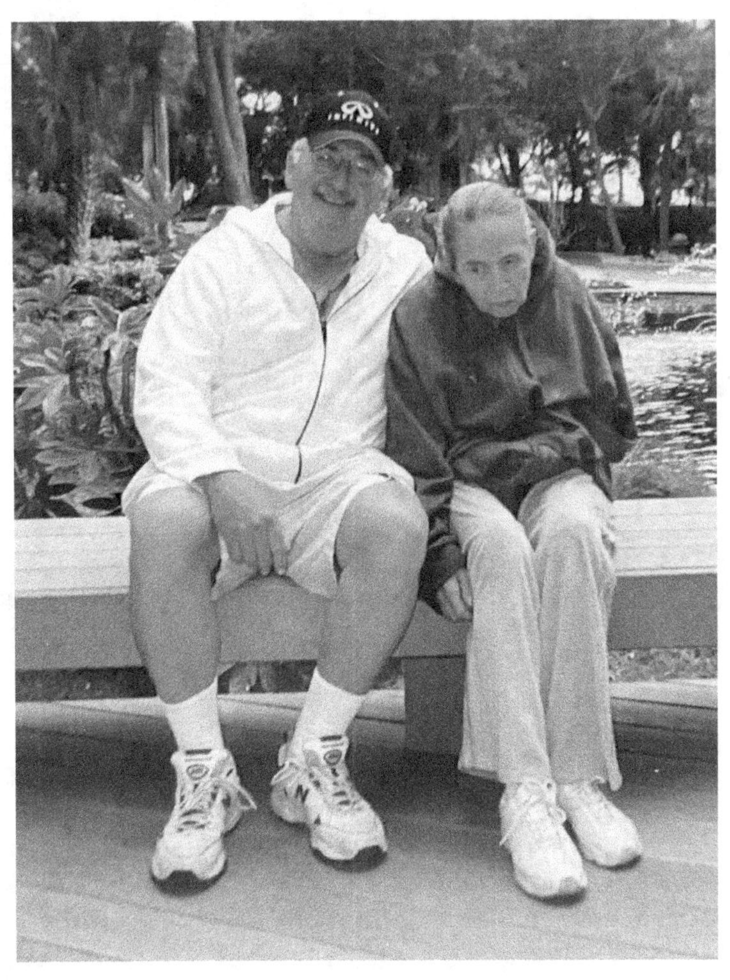

Elizabeth and me at Hilton Head 2007.

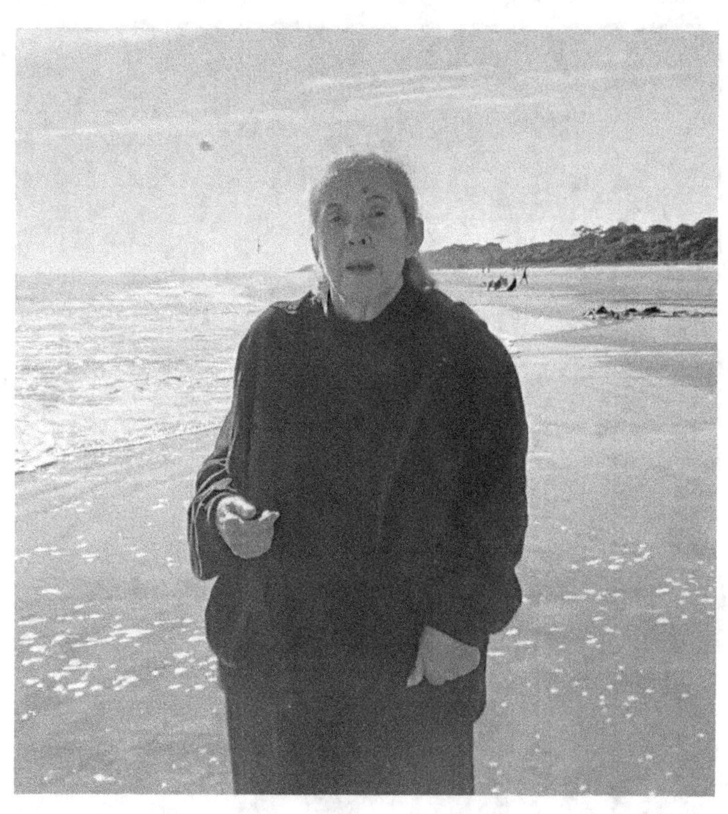

Elizabeth in ocean at Hilton Head SC

2007.

Chapter Six:
Funny Stuff

I don't want to leave the reader with the impression that my life as a caregiver was pure drudgery. There were frequent pleasant compensations.

You will remember that she had no filters to tell her what was appropriate, and so, in many respects, she acted like the innocent, guileless little girl, which could be cute, embarrassing, and mortifying all at once. As I grew more accustomed to her peculiarities, I became more hardened to embarrassment and more able to enjoy a good laugh.

There, of course, were the ads for free shipping and free gifts if you signed up for a credit card or a magazine. As a result, we were the proud recipients of more than thirty magazines and 20+ credit cards (before 2008, when credit was easy, she was always pre-approved for any number of credit cards). We were getting more magazines than my doctor's office.

Our daily mail was more than that of most commercial businesses, and we had no room for all the ridiculous free gifts we were receiving. I only realized how much trouble we were in when I confronted her with this question: "Would you purchase two elephants from the Bronx Zoo if there were free shipping?"

When she paused to consider it, I realized just how much trouble we were in.

There was a time when we were in Florida, and she needed emergency dental assistance. I took her to the nearest walk-in dental clinic, and we were told that as a walk-in, she would be waiting approximately one and one-half hours. I asked her to wait while I ran some errands and told her that I would be back before her office visit with the dentist. She seemed fine, and so I left.

When I returned about forty-five minutes later, I found my wife sitting on a stone partition in the parking lot, smoking a cigarette. I questioned her as to why she wasn't waiting inside when she matter-of-factly said, "They threw me out, and I am not allowed back in."

I was stunned! I went inside to speak to the receptionist, and she confirmed what my wife told me. She said that your wife was disruptive. She kept asking to use the bathroom, like every 5 minutes, and when she went, she passed the office where the dentist was treating the patient. She kept asking the dentist to hurry up and see her because she was tired of waiting.

After she did this several times, the dentist, not knowing that she had dementia or not caring, asked the receptionist to put her out of the office and to call the police if she resisted. The receptionist told me that the police were on their way and there was no way that the dentist would see Elizabeth, even if I returned to calm her. We quickly left before the police arrived and found another walk-in clinic. This time, I stayed with her the whole time.

Every year, our family business would win a free trip for being a top dealer for a certain manufacturer. This manufacturer would take his top 10 dealers in the world every year to Portugal, Spain, Puerto Rico, Bahamas, Mexico, Hawaii, etc.

This particular year, the free trip was a working vacation, seminar, and company meeting in Lisbon, Portugal. As I mentioned previously, my wife Elizabeth had a bad habit of excusing herself to go to the bathroom but felt she must tell everyone why she was going and what she was going to do once she got there. As much as I and other family members encouraged her to refrain from this behavior, she continued the pattern, seemingly enjoying the fact that it made us all uncomfortable.

Before the trip this year, I told her that I couldn't take her because she would embarrass me and the company we represent if she came. She promised that she would be on her best behavior and that she would not mention bodily functions when excusing herself to go to the bathroom. She wanted to go so badly and swore to be on her best behavior, so I hesitantly relented and agreed.

During the course of the trip and seminar, there was always a time to thank each dealer representative personally for the good sales work done in the past year. Traditionally, this was accomplished by being invited to dine one-on-one with the president and his wife. The day I received the call that we were invited to dinner, I was alarmed.

"What if you did something embarrassing?" I asked Elizabeth to remember her promise about "the bathroom situation" and to re-commit to her promise to behave. She did, and I felt fairly confident going into our dinner meeting that things would be alright.

During the course of the dinner, Elizabeth announced that she needed to use the bathroom, all the while looking directly at me and smiling, letting me know that she got it right. I smiled back, letting her know that I was proud of her for keeping her word. She soon returned, and dinner proceeded without a hitch. After dinner, John, the manufacturer's president, suggested an after-dinner walk. It was a perfect summer night, and a walk would be a marvelous idea. What followed was magical. It was as if scripted from a movie set.

The moon was out; there was a summer breeze. There was a man playing the guitar on a street corner across from the harbor. The women were mending the fishing nets broken by the day's catch and fixing them for tomorrow when their men again would go out in ships plowing the sea in quest of its bounty. It was such a romantic scene, and I was completely caught in a reverie. Elizabeth broke the reverie with the pronouncement that she needed to go to the bathroom again.

Of course, had I been thinking, I should have just let her go without comment, but I wasn't thinking, so I made a fatal error in judgment and said, "But you just went to the bathroom."

That's when she replied calmly, "Yes, but then I had to take a piss, and now I have to take a sh—t!"

She walked toward the ladies' room and left me with John and his wife. I finally said, "You know my wife is sick."

They said, "Yes, Fred, we have known it for a long time."

Sometime after that incident, we took what was to be our last plane trip together. It was late winter. We owned a condo in Florida, but we hadn't been there for quite a while. Elizabeth loved Florida. She used to call it her Bermuda USA. This was because both Bermuda and Florida unabashedly used pastel colors outside of their homes, giving them a real tropical look. She was delighted when I suggested that we go.

Also, at that time, I was starting to experience chronic backache, so I warned her not to pack more than she could carry through the airports. She was in the habit of packing lots of religious books like study bibles, and her bags often felt like they were packed with bricks. She also, as you will remember, was fond of throwing her bags down staircases.

So, when we went to Florida, I had my reservations and misgivings about what might occur. The morning of our departure, she started by tossing her suitcase down the stairs.

Okay, I thought, *let's just let it go. You can't complain about every little thing that's going to happen. Okay, she's a little odd; just deal with it and try to enjoy yourself.*

A driver took us to the airport, and we got a JetBlue flight to West Palm. We rented a car and drove 60 miles north to our place in Vero Beach. We were ready to start a week's vacation. My cousin Frank and his wife Clare lived nearby, and we made a date with them on several occasions to have dinner. We also contacted my old golfing buddy to play a couple of rounds with him and his wife, Sharon.

Everything seemed fine until my cousin dropped the "bomb." He came over one night with a series of cat scans and X-rays and clinically set them out for scientific study. He and Clare were both nurses, so I knew something was wrong if they were showing me, a layman, the X-rays. He showed me the film and pointed out some dark spots, which he said very clinically and devoid of emotion were cancer. He then told us that these were X-rays of his lungs and that he, in fact, had lung cancer. I couldn't believe it since he never smoked.

He said that he had contracted it by his exposure to Agent Orange when he was in Vietnam. He had been an Air Force medic whose job it was to evacuate the wounded from the field of battle. He had flown many missions through battlefields defoliated by chemicals such as Agent Orange, and his constant exposure made him a likely candidate for lung cancer. He was just starting his struggle with the cancer and was very hopeful he would beat it. He had the best doctors, all from Sloane Kettering, and he was in great physical shape and had a great attitude. We had dinner with him and Clare four or more times while we were there. Elizabeth was true to form and using the bathroom every few minutes.

At one point, Clare followed her to the bathroom and came back to the table to report that Elizabeth went in the bathroom, walked around, looked in the mirror, and walked out. She had no intention of using the bathroom. I thought immediately of something I had read about Alzheimer's and related dementias.

When a person with dementia is away from home or in a place where they are not totally accustomed, they get very nervous, and this can manifest in many ways. I remember that one of the ways was walking back and forth to the bathroom in a new or strange setting so you could memorize it in case you needed it later on. Except for my cousin's stunning news, the trip was relaxing and uneventful.

As we packed to return to New York, I reminded her not to overpack. I told her I had a bad back and could only carry my own bags. When it was time to leave, she once again let the bags go down the stairs, except the steps in Florida were concrete and might inflict real damage on her suitcases. We packed the bags into the rental car and headed off to the airport. We arrived, returned the car, and proceeded to the terminal, all without incident.

Once there, Elizabeth started to complain that she couldn't carry her bags and that they were too heavy. This, of course, infuriated me as I had painstakingly told her repeatedly (ad infinitum) not to pack more than she could carry. She stood there like a child, refusing to move unless I took her bags, which I knew by now were weighted down with books. I had no choice but to take her bags and let her take mine if we were going to make our flight.

We proceeded through security and all the way to the boarding gate without incident, but unluckily for us, there was a random check being performed by airport personnel right at the boarding gates in the presence of highly armed soldiers in camouflage uniforms. They singled out my wife for this purpose and started by asking those routine questions that most of us who fly have heard and committed to memory: **"Is this your bag? Did you pack it yourself? Did anyone give you something to put in the bag that is not yours?"**

My poor wife got caught on the first question. To, "Is this your bag?" she calmly said, "No." Offering no explanation or embellishments.

Upon hearing her say that the bag she was carrying was not hers, the security guards and the soldiers were startled. They weren't expecting her deviant answer and probably hadn't heard anything that shocking in weeks. The stunned soldiers raised the automatic weapons and were now pointing them at us. The security guard then asked her whose bag it was.

She turned slowly in my direction, pointed at me, and said, "It's his bag."

Now, all the automatic weapons were pointed **at me!!!** I smiled and quickly tried to explain the situation to the guards and the soldiers, to no avail. Before I knew it, they were doing a full-body search. Finally, after much security protocol, I was able to explain the situation to them. The humorless guards finally released us to fly, but with a strict warning never to do this again. Contrite and embarrassed, I vowed that this would be our last plane trip.

Then, there was our last **night at the opera**. Elizabeth and I had subscriptions for many years to the Metropolitan Opera and the New York Philharmonic. We always enjoyed our night out and a lovely dinner. This was the late winter of 2004, and the Met had the Russian national opera company perform Borodin's Prince Igor. The music is melodic and contains a wonderful ballet sequence called the Polivetsian Dances. This was a special occasion, so I booked dinner reservations at the Grand Tier Restaurant, one of the truly elegant restaurants in New York, right in the Metropolitan Opera House.

We enjoyed a lovely dinner before the opera's opening act. Elizabeth, true to form, asked the waiter for a take-out bag after she had finished less than half the food. Then, she started to pester me about whether or not I was also finished with dinner so we could leave. Of course, at the prices I was paying for the dinner, I was looking to enjoy a very slow and relaxing dinner. We had certainly arrived early enough so that rushing was not to be a problem. How many times had she ruined my enjoyment of a meal by rushing me because she was finished? The difference tonight is that I learned my lessons well.

This time, I was prepared! I deflected her readiness to leave by reminding her of dessert. I said, "They have a baked Alaska on the menu."

I knew she would love it and would want it. I also knew that before I got the waiter, and before he brought it to her, and before she ate it, I would have enjoyed the rest of my dinner in peace. I would have my dessert during the intermezzo when the restaurant typically served coffee and dessert to the people who wanted their coffee and desserts later. So, she said yes, and everything seemed to be going according to plan.

As the waiter brought the beautifully presented dessert, I was just finishing my wonderful meal. The baked Alaska was in the center of a large plate, and swirls of chocolate and raspberry sauce streamed off the top of the baked Alaska in all directions. It was a work of art for which the pastry chef could be proud. Elizabeth quickly finished all she wanted and was looking for the waiter. I realized that she was going to ask her to wrap it up like she had for her meal. I told her that you couldn't wrap ice cream and that it would melt in the car.

She, of course, argued that you could bag the ice cream and that it would keep just fine. So, as the waiter approached, I lowered my voice and told her unequivocally that she was not taking the ice cream home. She looked curiously at me, and then, faster than I could react, she lifted the ice cream, which by this time was melting all over the plate, and offered it to the two women sitting next to us. Their shock was great, and they moved visibly and uncomfortably away from her in a hurry.

Elizabeth simply told them, "Here, why don't you have this ice cream? I didn't eat much, and so there is no reason to waste it."

The shock and horror on their faces, and from their perspective rightly earned, would have, in the past, caused me great embarrassment, but now left me only laughing, seeing the hilarity of the situation. While it was quite funny, I realized that I could not put Elizabeth in this kind of position again. Once again, another chapter in our lives was closing.

Chapter Seven:
Starting to Get Sick

It was early winter of 2004 when I started getting frequent cases of indigestion, stomach and chest pain, back problems, and a general malaise that I just couldn't place. I just knew that I didn't feel well, and I was anxious all the time. I was becoming a nervous wreck.

Elizabeth had gained a tremendous amount of weight the year before, going from 130lbs to 195lbs. I really didn't care because eating was the only thing to which she still looked forward, and it seemed to give her a measure of comfort and pleasure. I wasn't concerned for her looks and health because we were dealing with a mental disease that far outweighed these small concerns. **My real concern became how I could go to work every day, not knowing what she would do when I was away.** The numerous episodes I discussed previously made me keenly aware of the danger.

One night a winter before, I came home, and my neighbor told me that an ambulance had taken my wife to the hospital. She was coming out of the car and slipped on the ice. She didn't get up but just lay there until the neighbor saw her. The neighbor saw the frozen hands and face and figured that Elizabeth had to have been out in the weather for hours. She called an ambulance, she said. I thanked her and went to the emergency room, where Elizabeth was being treated for hypothermia.

That year, while on vacation, I discovered a local chapter of the Alzheimer's Foundation and respite services and went in. The local volunteer gave me pamphlets that contained the National Hotline number. Now, in 2004, a year later, I was finally ready to call for help. They sent me a list of local Long Island, NY chapters.

After several telephone inquiries, I was led to the Long Island Alzheimer's Foundation (LIAF), which is headquartered in Port Washington. They (unlike the Alzheimer's Association, which looked for cures for this disease) were focused on resources for the caregiver. They had lists of support groups and respite services available to caregivers so they wouldn't feel overwhelmed and all alone. They gave me a support group in Mineola, NY, run by "JASA." I went there but quickly realized that it did not address my needs. This group was a support group for caregivers working with Alzheimer's patients, but invariably, these patients were either parents or siblings.

No one except for me was dealing with a spouse with dementia. That was natural because early onset Alzheimer's was relatively rare, and most Alzheimer's caregivers were dealing with older people, not people in their forties and fifties. Because they weren't dealing with spouses with Alzheimer's, they were not addressing spousal issues, which are vastly different from loss issues involved with parents and siblings. As a spousal caregiver, I was dealing with the loss of a best friend and lover; I was dealing with loss, betrayal, and abandonment issues, real or imaginary.

I then found the "Well Spouse Foundation," a national support group provider whose motto is, **"When One Spouse Is Sick, Both Spouses Need Help."** I continued to attend that group for several years, even though I was the only one caring for a spouse with Alzheimer's. Most were caring for spouses with other terminal diseases like cancer, MS, etc.

At least here, I felt like I could discuss the emotions of the loss of a best friend and lover. I went to monthly meetings, but they weren't nearly enough to get me through the stress I was under. So,

I found another group that met at the Bristal Assisted Living in East Meadow, NY. They had weekly meetings, and most of the caregivers were dealing with spouses, so I remained in both groups.

I still needed to address the issue of leaving her alone when I was at work. I did not know that respite services were available, some at cost and some free; some even sponsored by the county and by the various townships. Someone at the Bristal mentioned that Sid Jacobson Jewish Community Center had a respite program called the "Friendship Circle" and that they would take your spouse from 9 am to 3 pm if your spouse was accepted and after an interview and evaluation by one of the program's directors.

So, I called the center and spoke to Connie Wasserman, program director of the "Friendship Circle." She agreed to come to my home and evaluate Elizabeth for the program. Although Elizabeth was both antagonistic and defensive to most of Connie Wasserman's questions, which were designed to draw Elizabeth out a little, Connie decided that Elizabeth would fit into the program. I was thrilled and delighted as this would give me the ability to go to work, even if just on a shortened schedule. This was the answer to my prayers.

Because of Elizabeth's opposition to the idea (she thought it unnecessary and a waste of time since, as she declared, there was nothing wrong with her and we should all just leave her alone), Connie called me to the side and told me just to get Elizabeth there, and they would do the rest. She said that she and her staff had dealt with this attitude many times and that she knew if I could somehow get her into the program, she and her counselor would handle Elizabeth's transition to the program until she was happy to be part of it. I agreed to try it for three days a week to start.

The first day when I took her to the Friendship Circle, she was defensive and skeptical. She did not like the fact that most of the other "circle participants" were very old while she was only in her late fifties. Connie immediately picked up on this objection and asked Elizabeth if she could help them with some of the old people. That "hooked" her because she was now a helper and not a member of the group. She, therefore, kept her dignity.

Also, when Elizabeth complained that the plants were all in bad shape and that obviously no one was taking care of them, Connie said, "Oh Elizabeth, do you know about plants because no one here does?"

Elizabeth was delighted because she knew so much about gardening and house plants, and she was about to get the chance to showcase her skills. Connie said, "Great, Elizabeth, you can help us with the plants, too."

Elizabeth loved and looked forward to the Friendship Circle because she felt she had a job there taking care of the "old people" and taking care of the plants. I suddenly realized how adeptly Connie had hooked Elizabeth. Seeing that she was younger than most of the group and having met and evaluated Elizabeth before, she had seen that if she approached Elizabeth as a volunteer helper, she would have a good chance of getting her to stay in the program.

As the reader has probably figured out, a little deception is a great tool for dealing with dementia, and it works a lot better than protracted arguments, which get nowhere and upset everyone concerned. On our first day in the program, I was told by the staff just to bring her, stay with her for about ten minutes, and then tell her, "I had some errands to run and would return for her soon."

I was told by the staff to come back at 3 pm to pick her up. They told me that if I stayed, she would just look at me, cling to me, and not engage in program activities. These activities include word games, current events, physical exercise, coordination training, etc. So, I stayed for about fifteen minutes and discretely left, leaving Elizabeth in the good hands of the Friendship Circle's capable and loving staff.

At first, when I asked her how she was enjoying the Friendship Circle, she would say she hated it, but when I mentioned this to Connie, she told me it wasn't true. She said that once there, Elizabeth settled nicely into all program activities. So, I went to see for myself.

Without letting my wife know I was there, I observed the program from a discrete distance, and I saw how well Elizabeth fit in. Yet, when asked how the day had gone, she would respond that she didn't like and didn't need the program and that we were wasting her time and mine. I realized that she was only saying this to preserve her dignity.

She still wanted to believe and have others believe that she was in control. She knew that she wasn't old and infirm like most of the people in the program (the Sid Jacobson Center had not yet started their Young Onset Alzheimer's Program, where their participants would have been much younger and more Elizabeth's age) and that she wasn't nearly as bad off mentally as most of the other participants.

Nevertheless, her desire to help the "old people" in the program and her love of caring for plants kept her involvement intact. Elizabeth, in time, grew to love and look forward to her programs. We increased them to 5 days a week from 9 am to 3 pm, and she started taking the Able Ride bus to the program by herself, allowing me to go to work without worrying about her welfare while I was gone, at least until 3:30 pm when she would return home. This helped me enormously to maintain my work schedule and not have worries about how Elizabeth was doing when I was out working.

In the summer of 2004, my stress grew and was reflected in subtle and strange ways. My work required me to go to customer's homes to sell them the product and services offered by my company. I noticed that I was becoming more and more reluctant to go to the homes of our customers. I was able to talk to them on the phone and tried to conclude the deal over the phone so as to avoid traveling to their homes. I had not yet heard the term "Agoraphobia" and didn't realize that I was developing all the symptoms.

I still needed to address some of Elizabeth's medical and surgical issues. She had been diagnosed with an umbilical hernia and needed surgery to correct it. I needed to coordinate the surgery by hiring a live-in nursing service person to help Elizabeth with post-operative care (helping her in and out of bed and in and out of chairs and toileting) until she recovered. I decided to have the surgery done in November of 2004 and hired a nursing service to start the day Elizabeth came home from the hospital.

All through the summer and into the fall, I was becoming ill. I had feelings of being overwhelmed. Even simple tasks seemed overwhelming to me. I was depressed with feelings of isolation and that I was on this journey all alone with no help available to me from outside sources.

No one seemed able to grasp my plight, and I got tired of trying to explain how I felt. Friends were becoming scarce. A lot of our friends felt uncomfortable around her and didn't want to see us. This was a time when I desperately needed a friend's support and instead was finding this kind of support harder to find. I felt desperately alone.

I was supposed to fly to Hilton Head Island for a needed vacation and respite before Elizabeth's surgery in November. I realized that I needed to cancel the trip two weeks before because I was so anxious that I couldn't fly. I had anxiety attacks, and I was afraid to get on the plane because I might have an attack and embarrass myself. I was getting more depressed because I felt disempowered.

Things I was always able to do were now becoming impossible for me. I had been a frequent flyer for years, and now I was terrified to fly, so I canceled the trip and got more depressed. I was in the middle of a stress-induced anxiety-depression spiral and was heading for a major crash.

The day came for Elizabeth's operation, and I coordinated the arrival of the nurse who would take care of Elizabeth when she returned from the hospital. I could have, and maybe should have, waited and hired the nurse's-aide when Elizabeth left the hospital, but I needed to know that she was "on board" now and she would stay at my home and learn from me how to care for Elizabeth while she was waiting. I needed to control the situation as much as possible, and because I felt that I was losing control over my life, I couldn't take the chance that anything would go wrong for Elizabeth.

Having the nurse's aide a few days in advance meant that no one could tell me, "I'm sorry, we won't have a nurse's aide for your wife until next week." I wasn't going to take that chance. The operation went well, and we picked Elizabeth up and brought her home after a couple of days. Elizabeth was in a lot of pain but soldiered on quite well all through the convalescence.

During her recovery, I had the nurse's aide help me with household chores. We cleaned out the closet, and took years' worth of old clothing to Salvation Army drop-offs. We took Elizabeth, when she was well enough, to the Department of Motor Vehicles to get a non-driver's license ID card, as I have previously mentioned. I finally let the nurse's aide go after three weeks, at a point when Elizabeth was well enough for me to handle again. She resumed her daycare programs at the Sid Jacobson Center. It was at this time that I started to talk to Theresa Franklin, a friend of my daughter-in-law's family, who was looking for a job as a companion. She had previously worked for the family as a nanny for two of my grandchildren.

I liked her but was not quite ready to commit. I still thought I could still manage on my own. In early December 2004, I was getting progressively more ill. I felt stomach pains all the time, no matter what I ate. I tried eating less and less, which was easy because I had no appetite. It didn't help! The feeling of being overwhelmed was growing ever stronger and more frequent. The stress level was at eleven on a scale of one to ten! I needed help desperately but didn't know where to get it.

It was then that I decided to call a family meeting to tell them what I was going through, to ask for help, support, and understanding, and to tell them that it wasn't long before I had to put their mother into an assisted living facility. I wanted them to know what I was thinking and planning for and why I was doing it. I wanted their reaction. I also wanted to talk to them about Christmas, which was fast approaching.

Both of my sons and their families came to my house in early December. I started by telling them that I was getting increasingly ill and felt the time to make a decision about their mother was fast approaching. They disagreed and felt that I was exaggerating. They didn't see their mother as sick as I did and felt there was plenty of time to decide.

One of my sons told me that he thought his mom should never be placed in an outside facility but should be ill and die in the family home. Nothing less was acceptable to him, and he was totally opposed to my wanting to place her outside the home.

I got angry and told him, "I get it! I am supposed to get sick and die taking care of her so that at my funeral, people will speak well of me and say what a good husband he was, even sainted."

I said, "This is not what I want, and this is my wife and my life and my decision, and that I wasn't campaigning for sainthood; I just wanted a life after caring for my wife, and if I did die while taking care of her were you two boys going to be able to care for your mother after I am gone?"

That's when they all got silent, and I said, "Since I have to be here and well in order to take care of mom, then I must do whatever it takes to keep me well because, without me, no one was going to be able to take care of her."

My daughter-in-law Carol said, "Your dad is right, and he needs a rest."

"Fred," she said to her husband, "you watch your mom one weekend this month, so your dad can get away to rest, and David, you watch your mom one weekend next month. Also, four times a year, your dad has to be able to go on vacation, so you guys will have to watch her during those times."

My sons recoiled from that suggestion and stammered that they couldn't take time off from work and that they had a family to take care of, responsibilities, etc. Carol simply said, "Since you are not willing to give your father the help and the time that he needs, you have no right to insist that he try harder and with no help from you."

I was so happy and proud that someone saw my plight and was taking my part. I think when she spoke, she was able to make them understand how difficult it was to care for a mentally ill person, albeit their mother, because it would require so much time, effort, patience, and understanding.

I then told them that I was feeling so badly and so weak that I couldn't do any Christmas shopping this year and that I was giving everyone money. Furthermore, I was not going to send out any Christmas cards this year; I was just too busy and stretched too thin to even consider it. I was feeling so depressed and disappointed in myself for having to admit this because I felt that I should be able to attend to these things.

In years past, my wife and I both did the Christmas shopping, and both wrote out all the Christmas cards. Now, I was alone; she could not help me, and with all the time necessary to care for her, there just wasn't enough time left to do these otherwise pleasant chores. I was also embarrassed to be admitting these things to my children. My children, who had always looked to me to "fix everything" and make things "alright," were now seeing a father who could no longer "fix" anything and needed lots of help.

We were at an impasse! No one was going to convince anyone of the rightness of their cause this time, so we agreed to call it a night and to "sleep on it." I felt terrible about the way things were happening and was searching for some way to get them to understand my predicament and empathize a little with my plight.

What I didn't realize then was that they were in their own predicament. They were our children who wanted everything to remain static. Mom and Dad are not supposed to change! They are supposed to remain "the parents," strong, powerful, and all-knowing. This revelation about their parents' failing health and vulnerability was very upsetting to them, and they needed lots of time to process this.

A couple of days later, I received a wonderful call from my daughter-in-law, Carol. She said that she had heard what I had said and that she had an idea.

She added, "I realize it is too much for you to do Christmas shopping this year. You also know that I love to shop. So, how about letting me be your personal shopper? You give me a shopping budget for each person, and I will find a gift within that price range. I will consult with you on what I find and buy it with your approval."

This was the answer to a prayer and, at the same time, the nicest Christmas present that I have ever received.

I thanked her and told her that we would work together on it. She then offered to take my telephone book and send greeting cards to anyone in the phonebook, which I circled. So, the same girl who came to my defense the other night was now offering to take the Christmas burdens from me so I could relax and enjoy the holidays like normal people. I thanked Carol profusely and told her that I was in her debt and would not forget this kindness.

As Christmas approached, I started to feel worse and worse. I couldn't look at food, and whatever I tried to eat bothered my stomach. I was getting more and more stressed as Christmas got closer. Finally, Christmas came and went, and I still was not feeling right.

Then, on New Year's Eve, I felt pains in my chest and arms, and having gone through open heart surgery 10 years before, I knew I needed to be in the hospital. I called my sons and my friend Phil, and they all accompanied me to the emergency room at North Shore Hospital. I called Theresa Franklin, the woman I had interviewed back in October to be a companion to my wife, and asked her to go over to my house and cover for me while I was in hospital.

With everyone around my bedside and Phil, who had brought a portable DVD player, we had a classical music concert from Europe playing. In that happy company, I settled in for a very long weekend. It must be remembered that little happens in a major hospital over a New Year's holiday weekend.

The chief cardiologist, Dr. Katz, was off and wouldn't be returning till Monday. It was Friday, New Year's Eve when I checked in and had to wait through Saturday and Sunday before a heart catheterization test could even be arranged, so the best that could be done that weekend, barring an emergency such as cardiac arrest, was to have the nursing staff monitor me and give me blood thinners until the Angiogram test could be performed.

Even though I was in the hospital, I felt strangely relieved! Just being out of the house and away from the constant caring seemed to give me more peace than I had felt in a very long time. I started to become cheerful and relaxed. I started flirting with the nursing staff to help cheer them up as they seemed none too happy to be working this weekend, stuck in the hospital while friends and family members were having a "merry old time."

We were all stuck together, so we might as well make the best of it. We would all spend New Year's Eve together and try to be happy. This thought made me happy, and I became determined to be a model patient. I never realized until later that the chief reason I was feeling so much better was that I had a break from the caregiving, which in my case had become desperate, and I had help and support to enable me to take this break.

The weekend passed slowly enough, but I was not impatient. I was getting some good rest and relaxation, visits from lots of friends and family, and lots of "TLC" from the nursing staff, who by this time had all become my friends. The guy in the next bed and his family were hilarious. He was also waiting for a heart test, but you would never have known it from their actions. He was over 300lbs, and so were his wife and brother. They brought him pizza and Chinese food to replace the hospital "heart-healthy diet" food that was served in the cardiac ward. They always offered to share with me, but I wisely declined.

Finally, Monday arrived, and I was told that Dr. Katz would see me that morning. The hospital staff wheeled me into the catheter lab and left me with Dr. Katz's assistants, who prepared me with valium, etc., for the adventure that was to follow. About an hour later, I was wheeled into the catheter lab, where a catheter probe was inserted into a major artery. This artery led to my heart, and with a few deft movements of the instrument controlling the catheter, it entered my heart chamber.

Now, I realized why they gave me the valium. There were myriad TV monitors suspended in mid-air, and they were all showing the progress of the probe as it wound itself into every area of my pumping heart, all of which was happening now, in real-time, for me to witness. Thank God for the valium! I was so calm and clinically interested in what was happening that if the doctors had advised that they needed to cut off my head and re-attach it backward, I probably would have found that interesting.

After studying the cameras for a long while, Dr. Katz looked at me, smiled, and said, "Your heart seems to be fine; I see no blockages. Your oxygenation is very efficient, and all seems fine."

He started to point to specific monitors to show me what he was basing his considered opinion on and seemed well satisfied that I was in no immediate danger. I, on the other hand, was stunned by his findings because I had felt so badly for so long and was sure that my symptoms pointed to my heart. I was a heart disease survivor and knew and learned the symptoms quite well. I knew to go to the hospital immediately if any of these symptoms arose.

So, I asked Dr. Katz, "Why am I feeling so badly (describing my feelings to him) if, as you say, my heart is fine?"

Now comes a pivotal moment in this story! Dr. Katz answered my question by   saying matter-of-factly, **"Stress."**

I replied, "Do you mean that just stress can cause all of the horrible symptoms that I am describing to you?"

Dr. Katz looked at me and lowered his head so that his surgical mask was so close to my face that we were almost nose to nose. He then took his right hand and, with his index finger, poked me several times in the sternum while he said these transformative words: **"Just stress, you say, just stress? Just stress can kill you, and it is going to kill you unless you do something about it NOW!"**

His poking finger was used for emphasis, and with every word he spoke, he poked me so I could not mistake the gravity of or the truth of the words he uttered. The words hit home, and as I left the hospital, I knew what I must do; it was time! I could put it off no longer.

Three days later, I had an appointment with the sales director of the Bristal at East Meadow. I had researched many of the assisted living facilities on Long Island and found that this, for me, seemed the best of the lot; the rooms were bigger, the place was furnished beautifully, and my support group met there, so I was familiar with the surroundings. However, I went on tours of several other facilities just to make certain that I was doing the right thing.

I would learn later that the beauty of the facility was not for the resident but for their families so that psychologically, they would feel proud they put their loved ones in a "nice place." I was not ready to consider the fact that Elizabeth was beyond an assisted living arrangement and needed a higher degree of care, usually given in the dementia wing of an assisted living facility. I could not place my wife in a wing of the building where everyone was old (remember my wife had early onset dementia, and she was comparatively young and high functioning—no walkers, canes, etc., and could feed herself), nor could I place her where everyone seemed much worse than she.

As a result, the sales director told me that Elizabeth could live on the Assisted Living Side of the building, which was beautiful, and take all her daily meals and programs in the dementia wing. She was to be given a two-bedroom suite with a large living room and a small dining area. She told me that when I wanted, I could sleep over and use the extra bedroom, or one of my children or grandchildren could stay there. It all sounded so nice and so easy, but I just couldn't bring myself to sign the papers.

Chapter Eight:
The Big Hideous Decision

After my hospital stay, I knew I had to make that dreadful decision. I felt so guilty and so rotten, yet I knew my health was at stake, and I couldn't keep her in my home any longer without compromising my health further. I told Pat, the sales director at the Bristal Assisted Living Facility, that I just couldn't make that decision. My whole body was shaking, and my nervous system was frazzled.

She said, "Well, you're the only one who can make it."

I responded, "I want to go to a hospital and stay there and be taken care of and let someone else make this decision."

I knew this was stupid and irrational, but I was furious and, like a child, just wanted it to go away. I didn't want to take responsibility for what I knew must be done. I didn't want to be the "bad guy" who would be blamed for institutionalizing his wife, but I also never wanted to end up in the hospital again, and I knew I had to do something about it.

So, I realized that this was a hideous decision, but it was the best decision out of a host of other horrible decisions. I realized if I got sick again, there would be no one to take care of Elizabeth. I had to stay well; I had to preserve my health. I had to stay well to take care of her.

Three days later, I went back and signed the contract for assisted living. All that day, a strange feeling came over me. I felt like a terrible burden had just been lifted from my shoulders. I felt lighter, energized, and happier. I had a smile on my face and had a lot more vitality. This would be short-lived, but I didn't know it.

I went home and told Elizabeth that I was sick and needed to get away for rest. I told her that since there was no one to look after her during that time, I would be placing her in the Bristal Assisted Living until I returned, at which time we would talk of her coming home.

The social work staff at Bristal Assisted Living advised me to just get Elizabeth in any way I could, and they would make sure she was accommodated in her new surroundings. I signed the rent agreement, and our rent didn't start until April 1st, but it was not until April 30th that we actually moved in because we needed to use most of the month of

April to buy furniture, glassware, utensils, etc. before we could move her in. I had my two daughters-in-law, my sister, Theresa, and my two sons helping me with provisioning her apartment. I was so busy with the "doingness" of the chores to get her apartment ready that I wasn't noticing the ever-increasing stress, strain, and guilt that I was feeling.

On the day before she moved in, I was carrying the last pieces into the apartment. I remember carrying her suitcase, and my back suddenly went out, and I was in tremendous pain. I could hardly stand, but I soldiered on until the work was done. The next day, May 1st, was move-in day.

The entire family (my two sons, their wives, and Theresa) was present except for the grandchildren because we deemed it too depressing to have them be part of it. So, we assembled at my house at 10 am and got Elizabeth ready for her move. All was in place. The apartment was completely set up, and Theresa would go and keep her company every day from about 11 am to 5 pm; that way, Theresa was there to observe her intake of both lunch and dinner.

She could also take Elizabeth out in the afternoons. I also realized that Elizabeth couldn't order from a menu, and because of that, we were going to have a real problem with her eating in the dining room of the assisted living facility. If a waiter were to ask her what she wanted to eat, she would simply look up at him and laugh. In the past, I would always be there to order for her. But here, at the assisted living facility, there would be no one to help her order. I realized that she would not be allowed into the main dining room.

So, I set it up that from 8 am to 6 pm, Elizabeth would take all programs and all meals in the lock-down dementia wing of the building called the "Reflections Unit." In that way, I could work with the nutritionist to select a week's worth of menu items for Elizabeth. In that way, she would not be called upon to make any menu decisions and/or to have to answer any questions or make any choices. Meanwhile, I could hardly move because of the frequent waves of back spasms that would overtake me. All was in place, and she was about to enter a new life at the assisted living facility.

We drove, as if to a funeral about three miles south, to the Bristal Assisted Living Facility and brought her to the director of the Reflections (dementia) Unit. I had told Elizabeth that I was sick and needed to go to Florida for a couple of months to recover. I said that we had no one at home to take care of her, so she needed to stay at the assisted living until I returned. I told her I would discuss the possibility of her coming home when I returned from Florida.

As soon as I introduced her to the director of reflections and settled her in, the rest of us left and went to a local Italian restaurant. It was a mistake; everyone was crying and continued to shed tears throughout the entire meal. The director told me that it would be best for me not to show up for a week or two so that they could acclimate her to her new surroundings.

My coming during those first two weeks to see her might set back the process. I agreed not to come, but it was very difficult because I felt so guilty for putting her away that I needed to expiate the guilt by visiting her more often. I ignored their advice and visited her as often as possible. Fortunately, she was making a better adjustment than I was.

Chapter Nine:
Life at the Assisted Living Facility and Road Trips

At this point, readers may be wondering, *Why Frederick did you not immediately choose to put your wife straight away into the dementia unit? And why did you choose to have her live in an apartment in the assisted living wing of the building when she was already fairly progressing with her mental debilitation?*

These are important questions, and it is hard to understand, except on an experiential level, how these decisions are made.

When one is first confronted with the horrendous decision to place a loved one in a nursing home or assisted living facility, the driving emotions of fear, anger, and guilt are powerful and often cloud one's reasoning.

You think that you want the best-looking facility to assuage your guilt about placing your loved one there and so that visiting family members will be comfortable with the atmosphere (and maybe think highly of you for caring enough to find the nicest facility for your loved one). Of course, the right decision would have been based mainly on the facility's ability to do the best job for your loved one, not the looks and atmosphere.

You think that your loved one is certainly not nearly as badly off as the people you see in the dementia wing of the facility (and in my case, that she was too young to be with a bunch of "old people"), and you won't sign the papers unless the facility lets your loved one stay on the assisted living wing of the building (at least until you feel your loved one has deteriorated to the point of needing to be in the dementia wing).

Of course, the staff and operators of the facility know this, and they play along with it. They know that you are not emotionally ready to accept the fact that your loved one belongs in the dementia wing. They know that you will not place him or her in their facility unless they agree with you that your loved one is only partially demented and still highly functioning in other aspects of their daily life. They know that in about six months to a year, you will see more clearly and realize that your loved one requires more care and needs to be in the dementia wing—but now, at least, you are in the building and the transition over to the dementia wing is easier than a placement from your home straight in.

As a matter of fact, you will start noticing that new visitors to the facility will start looking at your loved one just as you looked at the "others" when you first visited, and you can tell by their distraught faces that they think your loved one is much worse off than theirs (and you realize that six months ago **you were them**).

The day I put Elizabeth into the assisted living facility, I realized that I could not live alone; putting her away was hard enough, but I hadn't lived alone since I was married 30+ years ago. I was starting to feel anxious, and with my back issues, it was all starting to be too much.

When I looked at Theresa, my wife's companion, who was crying inconsolably and who now had just lost most of her duties as my wife's companion, I asked her to stay with me, to stay over at night and to be there every morning so I would have someone to talk with at breakfast. I told her that after breakfast, her job would be to go to the assisted living facility and be with Elizabeth for six hours a day (noon till 6 pm) so that she would be with her for lunch through dinner. She would then return to my home for the night and repeat the routine again the next day.

I was starting to feel ill again. I was very anxious all the time; I was weak and depressed, and my back was getting worse by the day. I was sure I needed a new mattress, a massage, a chiropractor, a neurologist, etc. Something was gravely wrong with me. I started to "catastrophize." I was sure I had some kind of rare disease or maybe brain cancer.

So, I went to my family MD, who sent me for a brain cat scan, an orthopedic doctor for my back, an MRI, and a neurologist. I went for massages at the NY College of Physical Therapy, and they weren't working. I went for *amma* massages at holistic medicine institutes and for alternative therapies. I still wasn't getting any better. I went to the neurologist who ordered the brain scan, and I went to Dr. John Sarno (who wrote a famous book on healing back pain) for an evaluation.

After weeks in Dr. Sarno's care, it was decided that I needed to see a psychologist to deal with emotional issues affecting my back. This was a breakthrough for me because I was starting to see how much my emotions were being suppressed by me.

I was suffering from extreme anxiety and didn't even realize it. Dr. Sarno so often said, **"Learn to**

deal with your emotions, or your emotions will surely deal with you."

I also bought a self-improvement CD course entitled *Getting Rid of Anxiety/Depression* by Lucinda Basset. I heard her on TV and radio for weeks. Finally, I was so desperate that, even though I thought this could be just another phony claim, I was willing to suspend all disbelief and plunk down $450 to try it out. I figured the money wasn't the problem, but the anxiety was. I called and ordered the course.

I started with Dr. Sarno, the psychologist, and the Lucinda Bassett course in June 2005. I took an "all in, full-court press" approach. I decided that I was going to get well and that I was going to get well quickly. I needed to be proactive and work with the doctors to achieve the result we all wanted for me. I was going to take full responsibility for my problems and work together with the doctors to cure myself.

I wanted and expected speedy results, but, in fact, it took six months for me to drive a car any great distance and almost a year before I would travel by plane again. My way back from the abyss was a gruelingly slow process in which I really came to know myself as never before.

Meanwhile, my wife was becoming acclimated to life away from home. Theresa was there every day with Elizabeth from 12 noon to 6 pm. I usually went for a couple of hours a day, five days a week. At first, the hardest thing was to say goodbye. She would always try to come home with me, and it would tear my heart out to see the sadness in her eyes when she realized she wasn't coming. The staff seemed competent, compassionate, and friendly, and they seemed to really enjoy their work. I noticed how much better they were at dealing with her illness than I was. I soon realized that it was their professionalism that allowed them to be better than me. They were not emotionally involved with Elizabeth's progress or regression and did not take any of it personally, so it didn't hurt them.

Finally, by summer's end, I had a family barbecue, and I picked up Elizabeth from the assisted living facility and took her home for the occasion. We felt that since more than three months had passed since she was placed, she would be fine with coming home.

Of course, there was the possibility that she wouldn't want to leave and cause big problems when I tried to take her back to the assisted living facility, but we had to try. The social workers at the assisted living facility thought it should be okay, seeing that a sufficient amount of time had passed since her admission.

The family barbeque went very well, and when the company was leaving, Elizabeth turned to me and said, **"I want to go home now."**

I was stunned by her remark. I was happy and sad at the same time; it was so bittersweet. I was happy that the transition was complete, and she felt that the Bristal Assisted Living facility was now her true home, but I was also so sad. A page had turned, and we could never go back again. **She would never be coming home.** She had a new home. The thought of it was staggering. **I had lost her!** My life as I knew it with her was over, and a new life was beginning, and it was scary. I was completely out of my comfort zone.

As we all settled into our routine of visiting Elizabeth at her new home, and as she started to feel comfortable in her new environment, I started to institute a "date night," a once-a-week night out with my wife that we started when we were young newly-weds in order to keep the marriage zesty. So, I decided that every Wednesday night, I would take her out for dinner and maybe a ride or a movie. She loved Friendly's, a chain ice cream parlor restaurant. More often than not, we ate at Friendly's or some Italian restaurant that she loved.

Sometimes, we would take in a movie. This proved pretty tricky as she would always make strange sounds, and people would always tell us to "shush." A couple of times, I was forced to leave the theatre with her as she was creating a real scene. On one occasion, however, I took her to see a kid's movie, *Nanny McPhee,* and she and the kids all had a grand time making noise and laughing a lot. There were also times at Friendly's restaurant when she would lock herself in the bathroom and not come out.

At those times, with help from the manager, Erika, I was able to go into the ladies' room, crawl under the stall door and unlock the stall, help her pull up her pants, and take her out. Everyone at Friendly's was very sympathetic to our plight and made it easy for me to take her there. In the summer, there were concerts in Eisenhower Park, and we brought beach chairs and sat out in the afternoons and summer evenings.

Of course, we would always finish the concert by visiting Friendly's. Sometimes, members of my Alzheimer's support group (whose spouses suffered from dementia) would join us at the concert, followed by Friendly's. My wife's companion Theresa would also take Elizabeth to the duck pond at Eisenhower Park. They would sit and talk (Theresa would talk, and Elizabeth would sometimes answer back, but that was to become a rare occasion). She would soon stop talking almost completely. This, a woman who had been a published poet with an enormous vocabulary, was at this point reduced to about twenty-five words, which she would slur as she spoke them.

She was to be in the Bristal Assisted Living facility for more than five years. During this time, there were date nights and vacations where I, with the help of Theresa, my wife's companion, would take Elizabeth to the Delaware Water Gap, Hilton Head Island, and her sister's house In Pennsylvania, as well as her best friend's house in Hemlock Farms, PA.

These trips were possible only because I had Theresa, a woman who could clean and bathe Elizabeth, and thus made it possible for us to travel, occasionally up to two weeks at a time. These trips became fun for all of us, but especially for me because I could sense how much my wife appreciated getting out into the open air.

Of course, it is possible that I may be attributing more to her than she was capable of (as many pet owners do with their pets), but I choose to believe that she knew on some level that things were better. She loved the long car trips where she could watch all the other cars passing and being passed. She was getting progressively more childlike.

In the fifth year at Bristal Assisted Living, I intuitively sensed that this might be the last year that she would be able to travel, so I planned a very ambitious trip, hoping that I could pull it off. I asked Theresa, her companion, whether she would consider accompanying us down to Hilton Head, Charleston, SC, and Savannah, GA. When she agreed, we started to plan the trip. I had a timeshare in Hilton Head and traded my two weeks for weeks at the end of October 2009. We would drive from NY and follow I-95 South, stopping along the way for food, bathrooms, and motels to sleep at night.

We arrived after two days on the road in very good shape and settled into a beach condo apartment with a handicapped-accessible bathroom and an elevator, all of which were necessary since Elizabeth, at this time, was starting to become very unsteady on her feet as well as prone to passing out with not the least provocation. We

85

went to the Harbor Town Grill for lunch, and we had a beautiful time.

We sat out on the veranda, watching the golfers coming up the ninth fairway. We ate a beautifully prepared lunch and relaxed in the sunshine, enjoying the mild weather. After lunch, Elizabeth fell asleep, and we found that we couldn't wake her. She had entered the beginning stages of narcolepsy, and we were going to have to get used to it because it was to become a much more frequent visitor.

After a while, when she finally awoke, we took her for a walk on the beach, where she would walk barefoot in the ocean. It was such a pleasure to see her eyes light up, almost childlike, when she felt the water on her feet. After a long and tiring first day, we went back to the villa for the night. That is when Elizabeth passed out on the couch. Theresa and I looked at each other, both thinking the same thought. Was she dying or already dead? We decided not to call an ambulance but just to wait and see. We were reconciled to her death, if that was to be. It would have ended on a high note as she had a beautiful day.

We didn't wish to spoil it with an emergency room visit, especially since they couldn't improve the quality of her life. I never felt as calm about a decision as I then did. I knew Theresa and I had done everything right, everything that was possible to make her life as good as we could. I knew we had put out a one hundred percent effort. We held nothing back. We had nothing left to give her; it was finished. We sat there for an hour in quiet reflection.

Suddenly, Elizabeth woke, opened her eyes, smiled at us, and laughed; she was back, and we were all ecstatic.

These deep sleep states were to become her new normal. She was now to be diagnosed with narcolepsy, a disease where a person falls into a comatose sleep state at any time and cannot be awakened until the seizure abates. While the neurologist never said, it was clear to me that her brain was very ravaged by her mental illness and that these seizures could be expected to increase as time went on.

On this trip, she started to experience difficulty in swallowing solid food. We needed to cut her food into small bite-size pieces for her to eat. Also, she suddenly was no longer able to handle a fork and spoon. She no longer had the coordination to bring them to her mouth. It happened so suddenly that it caught us by surprise. Now, we needed to manually feed her all of her meals ourselves. We noticed how suddenly her changes were occurring and how quickly we needed to adapt to the new situation. This trip would mark the last time that Elizabeth was able to feed herself.

We started our journey back to New York from Hilton Head after two weeks at Hilton Head, a journey of eight hundred fifty miles. Naturally, we were concerned and hoped no incidents would befall us during our road trip home. We were not looking forward to visiting the emergency rooms of hospitals during our journey and the possibility of long stays if she needed to be admitted to a hospital for medical attention. We could only pray that our trip would be uneventful. We were stuck and had no control over the outcome. We left on Friday, planning to be home Sunday night or Monday, depending on the number of stops we would need to make.

As soon as we got onto **I-95** North, Elizabeth was happy. She loved car trips, and she seemed to perk up. She paid close attention to the cars we passed or were passing us. She was fascinated with the car lights and the movement of traffic. She was, in fact, your perfect long-drive car companion.

After eight hours on the road and numerous stops for bathroom breaks and food, we arrived at

Chester, VA, where we would stop for the night. Chester is a suburb of Petersburg, VA. Theresa had a daughter in Chester who was married to an army sergeant major and stationed at Fort Lee.

Theresa speaks to Bernadette every night, but she hasn't seen her in quite some time, so we decided to call her after we got our rooms. Bernadette met us for breakfast the following morning, and she and her mother loved up "sweetie peetie" (the nickname they had given Elizabeth). Elizabeth thrived on all the attention the two women gave to her, and so in that good frame of mind, we continued our journey.

Our next stop was Washington, where we stopped at Lois and Uncle Tony Romano's home. This was always a favorite place to stop, and Aunt Lois and Uncle Tony always made us feel welcome. We visited for a while and were on our way again. We found a motel in Maryland that night. On Sunday morning, we hit the road again, and five hours later, we were back in New York. We realized that trips of this magnitude would never be taken again with her, and we thanked our lucky stars for ending so well.

After that, we would make a couple of trips to Pennsylvania to visit our friends, Arlene and Ken, and Elizabeth's sister, Fran. As she continued her downhill slide, it became obvious that only local trips to the duck pond at Eisenhower Park and nearby restaurants were possible.

Chapter Ten:
The Support Group

In 2003, while visiting Hilton Head, SC, I came upon a sign for the local chapter of an Alzheimer's Association's respite program. I had been troubled for a very long time as to how to handle Elizabeth's worsening condition. I used my vacation alone to Hilton Head as my personal respite from all the cares of being a caregiver. And here, in front of my eyes, was a sign for a program that devoted itself to supporting those caregivers who were dealing with loved ones with Alzheimer's disease.

I decided to go into the office to glean whatever information they had. A lovely and helpful woman gave me the contacts for the Alzheimer's Association in the New York area and told me to call them for the list of support groups and services in my area.

As soon as I got home, I called and received the phone number of a woman who ran a group in Mineola, a nearby town. I went a couple of times but found the group (as most groups are) with the emphasis on caregiving by children of their parents who contracted Alzheimer's. I felt alone and alienated from the concerns of this group as I was dealing with the loss of a wife, lover, and best friend.

My emotions and feelings of loss were much different from the struggles of having a father who wanders off or a mother who lives with you and disrupts your household with her dementia episodes. I felt my needs would not be met in this atmosphere. So I kept searching and finally found a support group that dealt with caregiving for spouses with terminal illnesses; it was called "Well Spouse."

The Well Spouse Foundation had groups all over the country. It had nationwide conferences once a year. It dealt with mostly terminal physical illnesses but certainly did not exclude Alzheimer's. I was the only one in a group of twenty or more dealing with a spouse with a mental disorder, although there were many dealing with neurological disorders like Parkinson's, Huntington's Muscular Dystrophy, etc. Even though I was the only one dealing with Alzheimer's, at least the focus of the group was the caregiver-spouse and not the Caregiver-children and relatives. We were able to deal with all the emotions of a good spouse taking care of a sick spouse and everything that it entailed.

I stayed a couple of years with this group and found it helpful just to be able to talk to people who understood. I boastfully told them that I would put my wife in a nursing facility before I let myself get sick from caregiving like a lot of them had. I also, like a couple of other men in the room, told the group that I would like the company of a female companion to take to the movies, a play, and a walk in the park.

Some of the women found it shocking, but most of the men agreed. After a while, I believe a lot of the women came around because they knew things were not going to get better and that they needed emotional support. Going out would be a respite and distraction from the trials of taking care of a person with a terminal illness.

Around the fall of 2004, I found the Alzheimer's support group in my area. It was a unique group as it was completely devoted to caregiver's problems dealing with spousal dementia. All participants have either a husband or wife who suffers from some form of dementia.

Yet, even here, in this new group, I am still the only one dealing with the **early onset** form of Alzheimer's-related dementia. The group met at the Bristal Assisted Living Facility in East Meadow,

NY, and we are all so thankful for their support. We meet once a week, which is also unique, as most groups meet bi-monthly. This group continues to be a godsend to me and most of its participants.

Most of us look forward to our weekly meetings and getting the kind of emotional support we need to make it through the week. Many of us use the phone as a resource, and we don't hesitate to call some group members when we need help within the spaces between our weekly meetings.

Through the group, we have had experts in the field speak to us on caregiving, what to expect, resources available to us, end-of-life planning, estate planning, financial planning, respite resources, etc. I strongly urge all readers to seek them out. You can only benefit from the information and support they provide.

Chapter Eleven:
The Inevitable Fall

In the fall of 2009, Elizabeth started to have episodes of narcolepsy, a condition in which a person can suddenly and without warning fall into a deep sleep. This was first noticed during our last trip to Hilton Head when she fell into deep sleep after eating a luncheon meal. It was to be repeated often that fall and winter. Also, during this time, her sense of balance was getting worse, exacerbated no doubt by the neurological disease from which she suffered. It was now the late fall of 2009, and we enjoyed Thanksgiving with Theresa. Christmas was just around the corner.

In years past, we had always celebrated every holiday season by going to the Milleridge Inn for a holiday dinner. The Milleridge was always decorated so beautifully for the Christmas season, with carolers in 19th-century costume. It was such a happy and festive occasion.

We made reservations for us that year as usual. We were seated in our customary place, the main dining room with the fireplace and Christmas tree. We sat down for a wonderful meal and entertainment. We were happy! I ordered dinner for us, and when it came, I carefully cut and diced Elizabeth's dinner for the ease of squashing it further into a sort of puree, or like Gerber's baby food. After that was accomplished, I started to eat my dinner, and Theresa and I took turns feeding Elizabeth her food.

After a while, Elizabeth went unconscious and slumped in her seat. We recognized the symptoms and knew that she had fallen into a narcoleptic state. The manager came over and asked if everything was alright. I could sense his discomfort with the situation. I explained to him my wife's condition and assured him that she was alright and would recover soon.

I was sure he was embarrassed for his customers, so I said to him, "If you would like us to leave now, I would. Do you have a wheelchair?"

When he said he didn't, I said, "In that case, we will leave as soon as she awakes."

I also assured him she was okay, that this had happened many times before, and that he needed not worry. He then left, and a couple of minutes later, I excused myself from the table and went to the men's room. When I returned, ***all hell had broken loose!***

In my absence and without my knowledge or consent, the manager had taken it upon himself to call the police and the fire department's EMT section to take Elizabeth out of the restaurant and to the hospital.

When I returned from the bathroom, there were two policemen, two firemen, and a stretcher, and they were administering oxygen. As I protested and said there was nothing wrong and that she was my wife and had narcolepsy, and I wanted them to leave, that I had it under control, they told me, "Once called, we have an absolute duty to take patients to the nearest hospital."

I screamed, "But I didn't call, and I didn't want you to come!"

Then, the restaurant manager came over to the table to say that he had called while looking very pleased with himself because, after all, someone had to do it. I never felt so humiliated and hurt by the total lack of sensitivity. So, I was left with no choice but to follow the rescuers out and to the nearby Hospital. My wife's companion, Theresa, and I hurriedly put on our coats and followed. I was furious and determined to call the restaurant's owners the following day to let them know how a very long-term patron of their restaurant was treated.

When we arrived at the hospital, we were taken to the ER department, where we saw my wife on a gurney, waiting for a doctor to look at her. A little while later, the doctor arrived and asked questions to establish a baseline for the patient. I told him about her episodes with narcolepsy and that what he was observing was her new normal. He told us it would be a couple of hours as he was compelled to run a series of tests on her.

By this time, she was awake and conscious. He asked her questions, but as she hadn't spoken in quite some time, I had to answer for her. After running the tests, he smiled and said he was releasing her to our good care and that we could take her home now and back to the Bristal Assisted Living facility. It was now 11 pm, and we had wasted 2 hours unnecessarily just because of an obtuse restaurant floor manager.

We had learned a new lesson! We could no longer take Elizabeth out to dine except to places where she was known and loved by the restaurant staff. Fortunately, there were still three such restaurants: the Majestic Diner, Friendly's, and Venere Restaurant. She had been known for years in each one of these restaurants, and the staff had watched her deteriorate over the many years of our patronage.

It was now December of 2009. We continued to take her out once a week through the New Year, but things were about to change dramatically and irrevocably.

As previously mentioned, the dementia patient's baseline keeps lowering and resetting at lower levels as they move from "normal" to oblivion. These times of change are hotly contested by the family and loved ones, who resist the change with a ferocity born of love and a passion to keep the loved one safe from a future that will inevitably be worse than the present. So, the family and loved ones go into a full-court press to prevent the change from coming.

Of course, this is impossible and illogical, but as humans, we are normal in dealing with this change. We resist it with all our heart, with all our strength, and all our might, though we know change will work its will, and our resistance will fail. We don't care, and we resist defiantly anyway because that is what we humans do. That is what makes us human!

That being said, Theresa told me that she would be undergoing knee surgery in February 2010, so I would have Elizabeth all to myself for the month.

Early in February, I took my wife out for our regular night out, which was still a once-a-week tradition.

We went to her favorite Friendly's restaurant near the assisted living facility. She appeared to me to be a little worse than usual, but I wasn't concerned because this often happened, and she would recover and reset at her old baseline. I took her home and kissed her goodnight. I was totally unprepared for what was to happen next.

I got a call later that evening that Elizabeth had fallen on her way out of the shower, suffered a head wound, and was being taken to the hospital. I got out of bed and rushed to the hospital to meet her and the doctors.

When I went into the room and saw her, I was shocked. There was blood all over her forehead and a deep gash. She stared at me and seemed dazed. She was obviously hurt badly but showed no sign of pain. Now, I know that in cases of severe dementia, the ability to feel pain is seriously compromised. Elizabeth seemed to be in that condition. The doctors were running tests with CT scans, etc., and were happy to see me because I was able to answer the questions that would allow them to build a profile for the patient. After several anxious hours and a battery of tests, she was pronounced well enough to return to the assisted living facility.

During that time, I went over and over in my mind whether neglect had played a substantial part in my wife's fall. Yes, there was only one attendant with her at her bath, and yes, she may have been looking away when she got the towel to dry her off after her shower. Yes, my wife may have been left standing alone (although they told me she was seated on the toilet seat cover while the attendant, who was trying to dry her off, reached for a towel). I was supposed to believe that she sustained that kind of injury by falling off a toilet seat.

In my heart, I knew it wasn't true, but then I realized as I ruminated over these things that it ultimately didn't matter. A fall of some kind and at some point was inevitable. A fall is what demented people do. Their balance and nervous system are so compromised by that point that they render falling a certainty; it is just a matter of time—or as the old expression goes—they are an accident looking for a place to happen.

She returned but seemed much more frail and unsteady to me, but as I am just a layman, not an expert, I deferred to my betters and tried to believe she would be fine. The next morning, I received a call from the head of Reflections, the dementia unit at the Bristal Assisted Living facility. I was told that Elizabeth would not eat her breakfast and could not walk without two persons' assistance. I told them that I would personally come over and try to feed her, and if by the end of the day, she still didn't eat, then I told them I wanted her sent back to the hospital until she was sufficiently recovered. When I got there, I was agonized by what I saw!

My wife was passed out with her face on the table and her food untouched. She looked so pathetic and so helpless that I wanted to cry. I saw that her condition had so deteriorated that death was imminent unless I took quick action. I never considered just letting her go. I just wasn't ready to stop fighting, but in hindsight, that might have been best for her; only God knows!

I immediately called the best hospital in Long Island and requested an ambulance sent to pick her up. I did not want her to go back to the county medical center as I wanted to give her the best chance of a good outcome by sending her to the hospital with the best reputation in the county, and that was North Shore Medical Center at Manhasset, NY. It had recently merged into a giant conglomerate and had become North Shore LIJ

Medical Center. It was affiliated with Cornell Medical School and, through that, New York Hospital and Columbia Presbyterian (now NY Presbyterian) hospitals. I was going to give her a good fighting chance by getting her the best medicine available in NY—that is what I can do—the rest was up to her and God.

She was admitted to the emergency room on February 2nd, 2010. She was immediately put in critical care. After numerous tests, they told me she had had a massive brain bleed and that it would be touch and go for the next several days while they fought to bring the swelling and hemorrhaging under control. All of her vital signs were very poor.

For two days, she stayed in the emergency room waiting for a hospital bed. When they finally got her vital signs under control, they moved her into a room. They administered drugs to stop blood clotting and avoid strokes. They administered drugs to bring down brain swelling and stabilize her heartbeats. She was still in critical condition, and there were several "code blues" called during the first two weeks. She had markedly deteriorated from her former baseline. She could no longer lift a fork or spoon. She had to be fed, and that was obvious to all who could see, except for the hospital staff who blindly and mechanically brought her three meals a day, placed them in front of her, and took them away untouched an hour or so later. I became furious and complained bitterly to the head nurse about it. She simply told me that there was not enough staff to handle the feeding of patients.

After a while listening to the surreal excuses being offered, I decided that I had to be there personally from 10 am till 8 pm every day to make sure she was fed and actually ate at least two full meals every day. Without the enlistment of family, I don't know how patients survive long hospital stays. During that time, her arms and hands started to atrophy, contorting into curled and gnarled shapes and becoming stone-hard and unmovable.

I started to feed her lunch, cutting all her food very fine and then crushing it into a paste before feeding her, as she was starting to have some difficulty swallowing. During that month, between Feb 5th and March 8th, I became a fixture at the hospital. I got to know all the doctors, nurses, and CMAs who were taking care of her, and I became a part of the care team. She slept many of the days, and I read many books during that month, sometimes reading aloud to her as she slept and rested.

All that time, Theresa, my wife's companion, had been laid up, recovering from knee replacement surgery. So, all the caregiving was mine alone. Her vitals started slowly to improve, and toward the end of February, she was getting well enough to leave the hospital. Doctors came in to tell me that she would need a stomach port and feeding tube before she was released. I was not yet ready to consider that step, so I sought another solution. I had the dietician examine her, and they agreed to do tests to see if she could tolerate a dysphagic diet, one based on thickened liquids and soft food that required no chewing and would be easy to swallow.

We scheduled a test. On the day of the test, it was found that Elizabeth could tolerate soft food, i.e., food that was crushed into paste-like mashed potatoes and liquids that were of the nectar consistency. I was told that as she got worse, the liquids could be thickened to a honey consistency to prevent gagging and choking. The diet plan was drawn up and posted for the hospital staff. I was there to make sure that the orders were followed and that she received the proper food. Very soon thereafter, the hospital's social worker met with me to discuss discharge and where to place her. She would not be allowed back into assisted living as she now required heavy nursing care.

Very quickly, in the next few days, I saw and interviewed at least four nursing facilities and chose one. I told the social worker who was putting pressure on me to be quick as the discharge had to take place as soon as possible. There is tremendous pressure placed on the families of patients during the discharge process, and unless the families are tough and willing to fight, it is easy to be "run over" and trampled by the process.

I liked the facility called "Nassau Extended Care." Two of the women in my support group had placed their husbands in that facility and spoke highly of the caring staff. On my tour of the facility, I felt very confident in the staff's ability to perform at a level where I could be comfortable with the care they would give my wife. So, I went back to the hospital and told the social worker of my selection. She said that she would do the paperwork necessary to affect the transfer and that Elizabeth would be on her way.

The next morning, March 5, 2010, she was transferred, and I was there to follow the ambulance to her new and what was to become her last home.

Chapter Twelve:
Life in the Nursing Home

Mid-morning on March 5th, 2010, Elizabeth arrived via ambulance at Nassau Extended Care. We were received by the admissions/intake department, consisting of social workers, dieticians, and physical therapists. After all the information was gathered and the hospital forms received, Elizabeth was brought up to the 2nd floor, a floor generally used for temporary placements. In fact, it was a floor used by people who, after recovery from some traumatic injury, were sent home.

I told the staff that my wife did not belong on this floor, and they told me it was temporary and only until a spot opened up in the dementia section on the 5th floor. I was happy to hear this since my choice of Nassau Extended Care was based on the recommendations I had received about the excellent care provided by the nursing staff of the 5th-floor dementia unit.

In the first couple of days, things turned bad really fast. Elizabeth started to weaken rapidly and would not eat. When I investigated, I found out that the hospital instructions for a dysphagic diet were being totally ignored. When I questioned the head day nurse in charge of the entire 2nd floor, it became apparent that she was totally unfamiliar with the term dysphagic diet. When asked, she told me she did not know what it was and that they did not provide it. I was furious. I told her that I was promised by the admissions staff that her diet was no problem for them.

In fact, that was the only reason that she could not return to the assisted living facility, as they had no ability to prepare a dysphagic diet option. The social workers at the hospital and at the nursing home told me that the dysphagic diet was no problem for them and wrote it into the admissions order for Elizabeth. Now, a nurse is telling me that she had never heard of this diet and that they did not provide it! I was beside myself. I marched off to the admissions department and saw the department head. She called in the dietician, the head of physical therapy, and the nurse practitioner.

While there was no categorical admission of fault, there was a consensus that the 2nd-floor staff was not ready to handle a case like Elizabeth's. They specialize in rehabilitation, where generally healthy people come after undergoing knee, hip, shoulder, or back surgery, or where people who are involved with a serious traumatic injury, like a car accident, come for a short period of time to learn mobility skills before returning home. It was, in fact, only the fifth-floor staff that specialized in patients with dementia, and that is where she needed to be placed.

Everyone agreed, but until space opened up in the dementia unit, she would have to stay where she was. The department heads all agreed to waitlist Elizabeth for the dementia unit, train the 2nd-floor nursing staff on how to feed her, and cooperate with the physical therapy department in setting up a consistent PT schedule.

In this way, Elizabeth would both get exercised daily and be observed and evaluated by staff so that recommendations for a proper "care plan" could be created. Time went quickly, and as Elizabeth settled into the new surroundings, Theresa started to come around. She was recovering from knee surgery, getting well, and wanting to get back to work. We got a call pretty quickly that a bed opened up on the 5th floor. We took it immediately and thus began the next chapter.

We were all very pleased with the care being given to Elizabeth. The P/T was great, and she was making great progress with walking, climbing steps, and eating, and it looked like she might make a full recovery. She seemed happy, always smiling, and all the nurses seemed to like her, which was always the case with her. Her smile was winning, and healthcare personnel were always happy to have her around. She seemed to make their days more pleasant. Her doctor and his office staff were always pleased to see me when I brought Elizabeth to her appointments (this was to change within six months when Elizabeth could no longer travel and the nursing home doctor became her primary practitioner).

Now that Theresa was back, I was able to go back to just visiting a couple of hours a day and not have to spend full days with her, like when she was hospitalized. I was very grateful for that. Spring came, and with the improving weather, we took her for walks in Eisenhower Park by the duck pond, which she loved. We started to go out to eat again and feed her only soft foods. Except for the occasional trips to Arlene and Ken's house in the Poconos, there were only local trips to the park and to local restaurants where she was known and thus tolerated by the staff.

Chapter Thirteen: Final Chapter

As the disease progressed, even simple pleasures became fleeting. The disease progressed relentlessly, and with each downturn, we needed to re-adjust to face a "new normal" and, with it, a lessening in the overall quality of life.

At this time, I started thinking about what I might do if my wife needed a feeding tube to survive. Would I have the fortitude to make the tough decision to let her go, or would I, for my own selfish reasons, try to hold on to her as long as possible? It sounded so harsh! Were they my real feelings? Did I have the right to let her go? I had the power by virtue of my power of attorney and my power under her living will and health care proxy, but did I morally have the right to make a life-ending decision? I knew there were so many strong opinions on the subject, but this was <u>MY DECISION</u> and no one else's, so it really didn't matter what anyone else thought. I was all alone in this decision! No matter what I decide, I will find both support and controversy about my choice.

Elizabeth was to live in the nursing facility for a year and a half. Most of that time was very good. She entered the nursing facility in March of 2010, and as the spring and summer brought warmer weather, we started sitting outside with her. The nursing facility had a lovely outdoor patio and garden. We took full advantage of it during those months, which was only slightly spoiled by residents who used the patio garden as a smoking room.

Smoking was tolerated, and cigarettes were rationed out to residents, perhaps three a day, but some residents who were able to sneak some in through family members were able to smoke more. The staff seemed to simply turn a blind eye to the problem. I was not one to complain, especially when compared to her illness; smoking by some persons seemed too insignificant to get "worked up" about.

During this time, my oldest son, Fred, came every Sunday to visit, bringing his children with him. I would always be there on Sunday afternoons, and after his visit, we would go out to eat, leaving Elizabeth with Theresa. Theresa would make sure Elizabeth was fed her dinner and would stay until the nursing staff put Elizabeth to bed. My youngest son, David, came less often, but no matter what,

Elizabeth always seemed happy to see him and his family. That next summer, we visited the Poconos once more to attend Elizabeth's sister's wedding.

By this time, Elizabeth was in a wheelchair, and her bones had contorted into a gnarled effect, looking like a stroke victim. At the wedding, Theresa came to help me with Elizabeth. David and his family and Freddy and his family also came with us. Elizabeth seemed happy but confused, and it was hard to figure out whether Elizabeth knew what was happening around her or not. No matter, it was the last time that the family was to be together while she lived, and it was good that she got to see her sister for the last time.

Soon thereafter, she started slipping again. The blackouts from the narcolepsy came more often. The pneumonia episodes also came with increasing frequency.

Then came the episode I feared most. It was in the summer of 2011 that she stopped eating completely, and I was faced with that life-or-death decision. I consulted with the staff doctor, who was very supportive of whatever I decided, but it was clear that I had to make this decision alone. I decided to put the feeding tube in as I could not bear the other choice of intentionally starving her to death. I prayed that she would go naturally, soon, and without pain and suffering.

By August 2011, the doctor and nursing staff approached me to talk to me about putting Elizabeth in a hospice program. The nursing home offered it, and she would not need to move. I remember sitting with Theresa and the medical staff, tears flowing freely from both our eyes as we realized that the end was near.

We agreed that Elizabeth should enter the hospice program as a way to get more individualized care. Summer turned to fall, and I made plans to go with my sister on a much-needed vacation at Hilton Head, SC. As the trip approached, my wife seemed stable, and I left feeling confident that Elizabeth was in the good hands of Theresa with my sons, Fred and David, nearby.

I left for vacation on Thursday, Oct 28th, driving from NY with my sister. We slept overnight in North Carolina and reached Hilton Head by noon the next day. We had just stopped for lunch when **"the call"** came.

The whole moment seemed surreal. I knew what was to be said. I had prepared myself for this moment and had rehearsed it so many times before—but now—here it was. I was frightened and expectant; all my senses were razor-sharp. I listened intently as the nursing home doctor relayed the news in a rehearsed but gentle manner.

He said that Elizabeth had developed a high fever last night, probably from pneumonia, and passed away just before noon today. I thanked him for all his efforts and his kindness to Elizabeth and me over the past few months and told him I would contact a funeral director to collect the body. I was amazed at how calm I felt mentally while I could feel my body shaking. I told my sister what happened as she was already seated in the restaurant. She showed no surprise as she knew that my wife's time was short. We talked calmly and made plans.

First, I called a local funeral director to make arrangements. I decided that we should stay the night at Hilton Head to rest from the drive. We would begin our drive back the next morning and get home in 2 days. I called my sons and asked them to notify family and friends. I asked them to be available to go with me to the funeral home to make the necessary arrangements. We did all the things that a family caught up in life's tragedies does, but I digress. The important fact is that she was at peace, and her journey was over; she suffered no more. Now we could grieve for her, remember all the good times, remember her. Now, she was for the ages.

Postscript

Soon after the funeral, I was thinking, *How do I move forward?* There was so much time spent on caregiving, and now there was a need to redeploy that time in another direction. There was a deep abyss, and that abyss needed to be filled with meaningful things; otherwise, I would be stuck "in place" and would not be able to move forward.

My life, which was so full of meaning as a caregiver, now needed to be re-created and filled with something new. This was both exciting and daunting. I was no longer in the comfort zone of my routine. I needed to re-think my life and make it new. I tell you this because you, the reader, will need to go through this process, too, and will face the same choices, dilemmas, and decisions.

Another book on this subject will probably be written. Suffice it to say that a good support group and a good psychologist should stand you in good stead.

Good luck and good wishes for you on this life's journey!

Appendix:
Caregiver's Advice

1. Be in Their NOW

Don't argue with them; you can't win; even if they finally agree with you, within 5 minutes, it's a new conversation, and this one never happened.

Don't argue, tell them they are wrong, or call them crazy. Accept what they say and understand that they are sick; this is how they perceive things. Accept the situation and ask questions gently to try to show them a different way of seeing something. Or just go along with them. When my dad started to believe that the nurse's aides living in his house (taking care of his wife) had boyfriends in the mafia who were trying to rob him, instead of arguing he was delusional, I pretended to call the police and asked that they watch his house at night. Then, I told him that the police would watch the house. He was happy and soothed, and an argument was avoided.

When my wife refused to stop driving the car, which I knew to be dangerous, instead of arguing, I disconnected the battery and disabled the car. I also enlisted a neighbor to call the Motor Vehicle Bureau and report her. In this way, it forced her to accept the fact that she would no longer be driving, avoiding an argument that would have gone nowhere. We got her to give up her driver's license by taking her to the Motor Vehicle Bureau, turning in her license, and getting her a new ID card that looks like the driver's license. She was happy; she put it in her wallet and believed she still had a license.

2. Don't Argue

Even if you win, it's a new conversation every five minutes. What I mean is that no matter what you say or agree to, it is forgotten in five minutes time. Five minutes is all it takes for them to forget the entire conversation. You will want to say that we just agreed to this, or we just spoke about this. Why are we revisiting this topic again? The answer is that they forgot the whole conversation. It is better to deflect and deceive. The car driving story is an example of deception, and the thermostat story is an example of deflection. Instead of constantly arguing with my wife over turning the house thermostat up and down, I placed guards over all thermostats that required a key to open the guard. In that way, I prevented a dangerous situation without another fight.

When traveling with loved ones with dementia, understand that persons with dementia find all new places disturbing and extremely uncomfortable. Expect them to demonstrate anxiety and act badly as you have taken them out of their routines. Routines are safe as they require no thinking. New environments take them out of their comfort zone. Their home and neighborhoods are known and memorized by them, and they provide no new challenges. Whereas new environments create a totally new situation, and old routines cannot be used to navigate.

You must understand this, make allowances for their anxiety, and act out and have help with you to handle any unforeseen situations as they arise. I always traveled with Theresa, my wife's companion, to take care of my wife as we traveled. She dressed, toileted, and bathed her wherever we traveled. She was with me to help my wife stay calm in new situations, as Theresa was the familiar figure to help keep some routines intact.

3. Get Help for Yourself

Get a copy of *The 36-Hour Day*. It's a must for caregivers and a starting point for knowledge of symptoms, what to expect, and how to take care of yourself. Caregivers often burn out and get sick, need help themselves, and cannot take care of loved ones any longer. So, it is up to you as a caregiver to keep yourself well and strong. To do that, you need frequent breaks so that you can go to the gym, exercise, relax, shop, and see a movie with friends. This way, you can recharge and be strong and focused when you are caring for your loved one.

Remember, you need a break!

The Alzheimer's Association is a national organization and has local offices in most cities in the USA. You must call the local or national headquarters for information about respite services for caregivers. They will have a list of services in your area. There are adult day care programs where you can place loved ones in safe programs supervised by trained counselors.

Between 9 and 3 pm, you can be free to do whatever you want or need, knowing your loved one is being well cared for. Meanwhile, you get to rest, relax and recharge. There are respite services that come to your home and take care of the patient while you get out and away for a while. You can exercise and go to a show with friends, all to let you rest, relax, and recharge.

Don't allow yourself to be a victim!

After you get over feeling sorry for yourself (oh, why did this have to happen to me?), recognize that yes, you've been dealt a terrible hand, and yes, there's nothing you can do to change that fact, **BUT** there is something you can do about how you handle the situation. You can choose to be a victim (poor me), *or you can choose to play out that bad hand better than anyone has ever played it!* It's a change that now empowers you to create an environment where you can be proud of the quality of caregiving that you are able to provide. *Play out the hand great!*

4. Special Financial Considerations

There are many financial considerations arising from caregiving a person with dementia. You must consider a power of attorney to act for loved ones who may not, in a short time, be able to handle their financial affairs. You must get the power of attorney before the person is declared incompetent to sign a legal power of attorney.

If you wait too long, you can no longer get a power of attorney, and you will need to go through an expensive court proceeding to be named legal guardian of the person and property of the incompetent person. This is a timely and costly procedure that can be only avoided if you act quickly and obtain power of attorney before they are legally incompetent and unable to act for themselves. It is best to start preparation when you and your doctor agree that a decline in cognitive ability is taking place.

You must see an eldercare lawyer as soon as possible to discuss all legal ramifications. Important things to consider are getting all deeds and bank accounts transferred to you as a caregiver so you will have the money to pay all household, medical, and care expenses in connection with the person's long-term care during the entire course of this illness.

There are Medicaid, Medicare, and other insurance issues to be resolved, outside or in-home care to be discussed, and "spousal refusal" if necessary. Spousal refusal is a legal term under state (not federal) law, which in many states allows a caregiving spouse to file papers under certain circumstances stating that he or she refuses to pay and support the ill spouse any longer. If the application for spousal refusal is approved, the state will, under certain circumstances, pick up the caregiving costs by either paying for nursing home or in-home nursing costs.

5. Dealing with Grief and Anticipatory Grief

Grief is something that all humans experience at some point in their lives when dealing with great loss. It is a natural process we all must go through in order to heal. I want to discuss the difference between the grief we feel at the end of a terminal illness, like cancer, and the grief we experience as a caregiver of a person with Alzheimer's and other related dementias.

When you have a loved one dying of cancer, they only die once. Until their actual death, you have the ***very person*** you love with you. All the things that made you love them in the first place are intact. Their personality, etc. Whereas with Alzheimer's, you grieve in stages. You grieve every time your loved one sinks from one baseline to the next one lower.

This monstrous disease ***robs the loved one of their very personhood***, their personality, their smile, their thoughts, their interaction with you. You don't have the person you knew and loved any longer; you have a shell of a person living and breathing in your house with nobody home inside that shell. It's a terrible thing to witness, and the emotions that spring up are powerful. And you must learn how to handle them for the sake of your own health and sanity.

With Alzheimer's, we lose our loved one in stages, and we grieve for every stage of loss when our loved one sinks from one level to the next lower level on the inexorable path to oblivion. It's like the **Cheshire Cat** in Lewis Carol's *Alice in Wonderland* when the cat disappears in stages: first, the tail, then the body, then finally, the head disappears, leaving only the *smile*, which eventually fades out slowly, too. With Alzheimer's, you, the caregiver, view the patient's loss of ability to make good decisions, to live safely alone, to cook, wash, and go to the toilet, to speak and communicate, to eat and swallow food without aspirating into their lungs. Finally, their immune and other bodily systems shut down, and death inevitably follows.

You mourn each stage of loss every time there is a loss of function and a new setback or decline in your journey while anticipating the final outcome. That's the definition of anticipatory grief: **EXPECTING LOSS**. I can recommend two good books on the subject of grief and dealing with it: *On Grief and Grieving* by E. Kubler-Ross, MD (*The Five Stages of Grief*) and *Expecting Loss* by Alan Wolfelt, Ph.D. Of course, I cannot overstate your obtaining and devouring *The 36-Hour Day* by Mace and Rabins, MD.

6. Join a Support Group

*I cannot **overstress** the importance of this step.* I was desperate and overwhelmed when I started to explore the possibility of joining a support group, and now, after 10-plus years of co-leading a support group, I see every new person coming into our group is both desperate and overwhelmed, seeking relief and understanding. You can't do this alone unless you are a professional caregiver, even then, because it is not personal to them.

For non-professional caregivers caring for their own loved ones, your objectivity as a caregiver falters and often clouds your ability to make correct decisions. I like the motto of the Well Spouse Foundation, which is **"When One Spouse Is Sick, Both Spouses Need Help."**

The support group is your port in a storm. Everyone understands your concerns, needs, and problems. It is a safe place to vent and emote as everyone has been there and understands. You can be assured that what you or anyone else in the group says is sacred and stays right there.

Many times, your friends or family don't see and don't understand the problems and stresses that you are dealing with constantly and on a daily basis. Only your support group understands and can give you the advice and compassion you need to deal with your life as it is now and in this moment. This is so true because your life can change instantly as you are forced to react to things that may happen suddenly and out of the blue. For example, when and if they wander and go missing, do dangerous things in and around the house or in the neighborhood.

Finally, the support group is a fountain of useful information on caregiving. They have guest speakers who are lawyers, doctors, or nurses who are trained in caring for dementia patients. There, you will find information on respite services offered locally.

As I said earlier, it is critically important for you to get frequent breaks from caregiving to relax and recharge. These respite services, whether in an adult day care facility or in-home service, allow you to go shopping, to a movie, play a sport, go for a walk or gym, etc., while knowing that your loved one is safe while you're away.

Here are some resources that may be able to assist you:

- Alzheimer's Association
- Alzheimer's Foundation
- Alzheimer's Disease Resource Center
- Long Island Alzheimer's Foundation
- Lutheran Counseling Center
- Catholic charities
- JASA
- Local government respite programs
- Sid Jacobson Jewish Center dementia programs (Connie Wasserman, Director)

These are samples of the downstate New York area. You will need to find out where similar programs are offered in your area of the country.

Adult daycare programs are offered locally everywhere, but you will need to find them in your own area.

The 36-Hour Day—an essential book and caregivers manual for caring for a person with Alzheimer's and related dementias.

Acknowledgments

Thanks to Connie Wasserman, the staff at the Friendship Circle, the Bristal, East Meadow staff, especially the Reflections staff, our support group members, and especially my family and friends who saw me through some of my darkest moments.

To suffer woes which Hope thinks infinite; To forgive wrongs darker than death or night; To defy power which seems omnipotent ; ….Neither to change, nor falter, nor repent; …..This is to be good, great and joyous, beautiful and free; This is alone Life,Joy,Empire and Victory

From Prometheus Unbound

By Percy Bysshe Shelly

About the Author

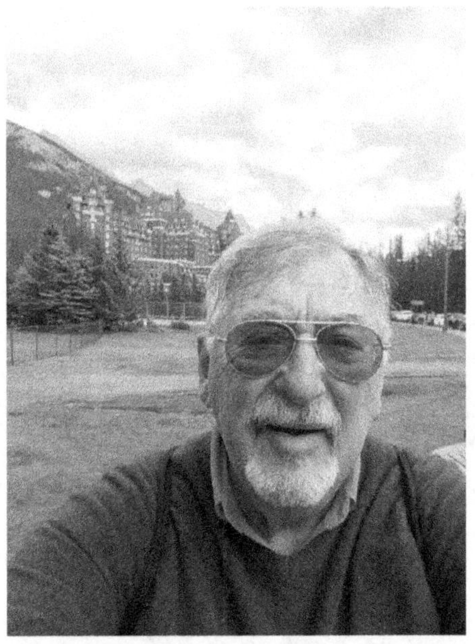

Frederick Russo is a retired attorney, company president, and teacher. He writes short stories, children's books, and poems as a hobby and has one published poem. This is his first published book, with others planned.

He resides in New York, near his family, and in Florida.